Borrowing Time

Borrowing Time

Growing Up with Juvenile Diabetes

Pat Covelli

Thomas Y. Crowell, Publishers
Established 1834, New York

FIRST EDITION

DESIGNER: LESLIE PHILLIPS

Library of Congress Cataloging in Publication Data

Covelli, Pat.
    Borrowing time.

    1. Diabetes in children—Biography.   2. Diabetes
—Biography.   3. Covelli, Pat.   II. Title.
RJ420.D5C69   1979   362.1'9'646209 [B]   779–7083
ISBN 0–690–01841–X

79 80 81 82 83 10 9 8 7 6 5 4 3 2 1

For CAROL,
who keeps me sane, alive,
and fighting

Contents

PROLOGUE 15

1. THE BEGINNING 17

2. NORMAL? 27

3. IMAGES OF DEATH 35

4. INVALID 47

5. A HEALING SUMMER 55

6. FREEDOM AND FEAR 63

7. THE ABSURDITY OF DEATH 79

8. VISION 91

9. PAINFUL STEPS 99

10. PERIPHERAL VISION 111

11. TILL DEATH DO US PART 119

12. EXTREMITIES 129

13. DEGENERATION 135

14. BACKUPS 143

15. UNANSWERED QUESTIONS 153

16. REGENERATION 159

Acknowledgments

To my mother, for literally keeping me alive through the rough years
To my father, a tough man with a soft spot, who understands and loves too well
To Ralph, Rosanne, and John, who have helped in countless ways
To Baby Lena, whose life reaffirms my faith
And to Freddy, who lived the same dreams, and who has saved me more times than he will ever know
I love you all.

I also want to thank those who have helped along the way:
John Cheever, for conversation and kind words in a city he abhors
Jed Mattes, for believing in a young writer
Susan Muldow, who helped plant the seeds for the project
Walter Meade, who gave time, encouragement, and advice
And Laurens Schwartz, for advice, fine prose, and friendship

Enlightenment comes to the most dull-witted. It begins around the eyes. From there it radiates. A moment that might tempt one to get under the Harrow oneself. Nothing more happens than that the man begins to understand the inscription, he purses his mouth as if he were listening. You have seen how difficult it is to decipher the script with one's eyes; but our man deciphers it with his wounds.

FRANZ KAFKA

Borrowing Time

Prologue

I HAVE LIVED with diabetes for fifteen years. This book re-counts my struggle during those years with the physical and psychological aspects of dealing with a chronic illness. Diabetes kills. It can cause blindness, gangrene, and a host of other complications. My main concern, however, is with the way the diabetic can cope and come to terms with his illness. Diabetes *causes* nothing but physical symptoms, yet I have tried to relay, through my own personal experience, how common fears can become intensified by their relationship to diabetes.

Diabetes is an omnipresent disease, and a degree of fusing of everyday concerns with the disease is inevitable. That is why I use the term "diabetic mind" in the book—merely as a point of reference. In no way do I mean to imply that diabetes is necessarily harmful to a person's psychological well-being. But it must be dealt with psychologically.

It is, in the end, what we make of it. I believe in facing the truth: not only the physical facts, but also the interior questions. It is my hope that this book will be of help to those who have to deal with similar questions.

1

The Beginning

I WAS TEN YEARS OLD and could not sleep. The sheets on the bed were a tangled mass, stained yellow with sweat. There was no rest: sleep simply would not come.

Several times during that night I got up, exhausted and weak, because my bladder seemed filled to the point of bursting. Urine spilled into the toilet in a slow, painful trickle. There was so much to expel, yet it came so slowly. The urine was thick and difficult to pass, and a burning sensation came with every effort. The damp, clammy cold of the bathroom tiles seeped through my feet, rising until my legs began to cramp.

I would no sooner leave the bathroom than the urge to urinate would return, along with the uncomfortable pressure of a filled bladder and the burning sensation in the groin. Trips to the toilet that night became a ritual—and still I could not sleep.

Something was wrong, I knew—not the demons of childhood nightmares, but something physical. As a child of ten, though,

I could not make any logical connections. I could only sense the presence of physical danger.

Innocence is rooted in the belief that all pain can be removed by the magic hands of a mother and father. A child's first experience of pain that does not go away, that cannot be soothed, makes him sense the terrible truth that suffering can become a way of life. He may fight against the realization by clinging to his innocence: the pain *will* go away. But instinctively he keeps the matter to himself, suspecting deep down that his world will be changed forever.

My own line of defense was to withdraw. I kept my mouth shut. My mother thought I was upset over the absence of my father, who was in the hospital. I prayed for him during the sleepless nights, for his warmth and comfort, for his strong hands and soothing voice. I asked God to bring him back home to us, to make everything normal again.

But in less than a week my body had become a siphon, with a continual stream pouring from it. The symptoms came in waves of horror: there was the unquenchable thirst, and the parched, burning sensation throughout my body. I remember a constant shuttle between the faucet, where I gulped water, and the toilet. My eyes would go out of focus. A simple cut refused to heal. Boils erupted on the back of my head and neck.

I began to lose weight, yet I was always hungry. Like a scavenger, I searched the kitchen for food. I felt as if I was starving to death. (In fact, I would later learn, I was.) There was always a peculiar, acidic taste in my mouth. And always the burning, the weakness, the exhaustion.

But what I remember most is the awful dread of a child who did not understand what was happening to his body. A child who could not know that he was close to coma and death.

My father came home from the hospital, and my faith in the mythic healing powers of parents was shattered forever: the God of childhood prayers no longer listened. Retreating to the basement, I stared at the smoked-glass panels with butterflies pressed between the layers, and knew there and then, somehow, that the sickness would never go away.

Now that my father had regained his health, my mother began to notice the light filtering from the bathroom so often during the night, the constant flow of tap water in the sink, my unending hunger, my hollow eyes. Finally, when she saw the pounds melt away, the actual transformation of mass and shape, she knew this was no ordinary childhood disease.

I believe I lost my boyhood forever the day we went to the doctor. I state it that way without regret or a sense of loss. On that day, one life ended and a new one began. This is said after a painful journey to the realization of just how powerless we are over many things in our lives, most notably physical disease. To fight this fact, to deny it, is deadly. I have tried, and in the process have damaged myself physically and hurt many others along the way. Only through acceptance of the unchangeable in life can a person begin to live.

At the age of ten, I began the journey.

I have relived the scene countless times, the memory filtered through the fear I felt then. I had never been frightened of the doctor before. His hair was slick, pure silver, and brushed back —the kind of doctor remembered for soft words, a comforting manner, a wide smile. His face showed the gentle lines of graceful aging.

I had the impression that my mother was talking about someone else when she began to tick off the symptoms: the frequency of urination, thirst, hunger, weakness, boils, lack of sleep, depression. Then it all began to come together in my mind, began to take on shape, however vague.

The doctor nodded his head as if he knew the answer. I did not want to know, had a terrible, unreasonable fear that anything he said would only make matters worse. It was the elemental fear of recognition: I somehow knew that a single revelation can change a life forever. If he said the words, then, and only then, would it come true. Denial of this kind is protection for a child—indeed, for all of us, at times.

The doctor asked me if I could urinate into a bottle. I needed little excuse to empty my bladder. He took a thin, coated strip and put it in the liquid. It began to change. I was transfixed as it finally settled into a dark shade of green. I thought it was some kind of trick, a game like the candy at the end of the visit.

The doctor frowned. "I think we'd better take him to the hospital," he said. "It's diabetes—juvenile diabetes."

He began to explain to my mother, but I didn't really hear him. The new word kept reverberating in my mind. A label, finally, for all that had been happening. I heard the word "sugar," but could not connect it with diabetes, the spoken word that would change my life.

My mother wanted me to see my father before I went to the hospital, but the doctor said it was crucial that I get there. I could go into coma any minute.

The doctor did not give me any candy when we left the office.

Thirteen years later, I laughed when I came across a term in a medical dictionary: *diabetophobia,* defined as a morbid fear of becoming a diabetic. I thought it amusing to find a trauma from which I could never suffer.

Diabetes is feared because it is not understood: the fact is that few people die of diabetes, but the complications of the disease are a major cause of death. This relationship cannot be ignored.

There is no precise medical consensus, even today, on what constitutes diabetes. It is, in many respects, an unknown disease. For years, all forms of its manifestation were lumped together as one disease, but many researchers now distinguish between two separate forms of diabetes.

The juvenile-onset type appears early in life, usually in childhood or the teens. The pancreas loses its ability to produce insulin, a hormone that breaks down sugar-forming foods so the sugar can enter the cells and be used as energy. Without insulin, the cells cannot metabolize sugar, and they—and the victim— literally starve to death.

So the juvenile diabetic must take injections of insulin every day of his life. Most people think that this solves the problem, that insulin is a *cure* for diabetes. Many doctors, on the other hand, are beginning to believe that it might be a curse.

The human pancreas is a marvelous computer; the injection needle, by comparison, a thoughtless mass of plastic and steel. A functioning pancreas knows when and how much insulin to secrete. After a meal, insulin secretion flows in the proper proportion. After strenuous exercise it slows, because the body is burning up its energy. If a diabetic runs to catch a bus, he will burn up sugar, yet the insulin he has injected remains at the same level. He might therefore have too much insulin in his body, which produces a dangerous reaction. If this reaction strikes suddenly, he can pass out.

Some infections can also cause the body's sugar to rise, and again, the injection does not take this into account. The diabetic is more prone to infection than a healthy specimen, and, psychologically as well as physically, his capacity to heal is reduced. It is often a slow and painful process.

Emotions, too, play a role in diabetes. Both tension and anxiety can make the sugar soar out of control.

Most experts declare that the juvenile diabetic can lead a "normal" life, usually qualified by the words "relatively," or "for some time." I don't know what a "normal" life might be, but I do know that the mortality rate of the juvenile diabetic is very high. After about twelve years, 80 percent of all juvenile diabetics develop blood-vessel diseases that contribute to a host of complications: kidney, liver, and nerve damage; arteriosclerosis; heart attacks and strokes. Poor circulation makes gangrene a constant threat. Diabetic retinopathy, which causes the blood vessels of the retina to burst, is a leading cause of blindness in the United States. I have been a diabetic for fifteen years, and have seen patients younger than I go blind.

The reality of these possibilities should not be buried under vague notions of normalcy. Diabetes is more than a physical disease. It is a long journey to the conquest of fear. I believe that awareness of the disease's complications can make a person live more intensely in the present, thus bringing a valuable perspective to all his senses.

The other form of diabetes, maturity-onset, carries with it some of the same problems, but most people who contract the disease—usually after the age of forty—do not take insulin. Diet and/or oral drugs are generally prescribed; complications are less severe. There are an estimated ten to twenty million maturity-onset diabetics in the United States; there are one million juvenile types.

It is believed that heredity plays a role in diabetes, and that a combination of genes, triggered by a virus, might bring on the juvenile type. There is a good chance that those with diabetes will pass it down through generations.

Doctors argue over these and other questions, the most

frightening of which is the one that springs from the recently propounded theory that insulin itself causes all the blood-vessel diseases. The theory is that injected insulin is too concentrated as it passes through the system on its way to the liver, and thus causes damage along the way.

\

That word; all those people in white running around and saying that word: *diabetes.*

My mother leaving, crying. I wanted her to stay, the only link I had with the world of warmth and comfort I had known for ten years, a simple life now shattered. That kind of trauma takes deep root in the mind, filters into nightmares and affects every waking moment for the rest of one's life. It is a moment the diabetic should never forget, because he can harness the experience and make his life more valuable. He can know the value of sight because he lives every day with the possibility of blindness; he can appreciate life itself because he knows that the simple fact of living cannot be taken for granted.

But the child only knows fear. My mother gone, I was now alone in that white room. After fifteen years I can still recall the frightening silence, a stillness broken only by that one word, the one that held such secret meanings. The weakness and dryness were getting worse.

Then a man in a white suit entered the room. He told me to lift my arm. He pulled out the biggest needle I had ever seen and tied a strip of rubber around my right arm. I closed my eyes for the initial attack.

He missed. I heard him mutter something under his breath as a thin stream of blood began to ooze down my arm. I felt a sharp stab of pain as he attacked for the second time.

Another miss.

To keep from crying, I counted all the times this man stabbed me with the needle. I remember thinking that he must not ever have done this before.

Six.

Seven.

Eight.

Knowing nothing about interns, I asked the man if he was a doctor. He did not answer. My arm was dotted with puncture marks and was turning purple. There was a good deal of blood spilling down on me, but nothing in the syringe.

I lost much of my faith in doctors that day. My loss of faith may have been unreasonable and unjust, but so many of our beliefs take root in childhood and are difficult to overcome.

I told the man he was hurting my arm. He just grunted, and it occurred to me that it was *my* arm, and what did he care?

Then he asked me if I was left-handed.

"Yes," I answered.

"That's the problem," he said. "Give me your left arm."

If that was the problem, it wasn't solved easily. "You have the worst veins I've ever seen," he said. My left arm was beginning to match the shade of my right.

Four.

Five.

Six.

Lucky seven; the intern hit it. He seemed quite proud of himself, not caring that both my arms were now sore and bleeding. The blood flowed very slowly into the syringe, and he kept moving the needle around in my arm. Tears were beginning to run down my face. I remember to this day that he did not offer me one word of comfort, did not even say he was sorry, when he left. A single kind word would have done a great deal to ease my fears. He put a Band-Aid on the successful puncture, as if by ignoring all the others he could deny their existence. I learned something important that day when I told myself that it was not *his* arm that bled: it was the beginning of the realization that each of us has a grave responsibility to our own body. Ultimately it is we who are in charge; no one in the world has more concern for a body and its welfare than the owner. No one.

I was alone again, but not for long. Every hour, that first night, a nurse would come in to take a blood sample and then give me an injection of insulin. One time a doctor came in and the nurse said, "Four hundred." Later I learned that this meant the sugar level in my blood. The normal sugar count ranges from 80 to 120.

That was my first night of a two-week stay in the hospital. The nurses tried to explain about diabetes, but I didn't really understand. They began to measure the fragile balance of my body's need for insulin. My mother sat with me during the day, and during the evening my father would come and feed me and make me laugh.

Slowly I began to feel better. One day a nurse came in to teach me to play a new game. What fun it was to stab those oranges with a needle, how easy it was to jab it into the skin with a quick snap of the wrist.

After two weeks I began to cry, saying that I wanted to go home. The doctor said I would have to give myself a needle before I could leave; I was willing to try. So I snapped the covers from both ends of the syringe and put them on the table. I eased the plunger back and forth slowly, then pierced the rubber stopper of the vial with the thin sliver of steel. With a quick motion, I pulled the plunger back, drawing the milky substance into the syringe, then pushed back to expel the air bubbles.

I aimed the needle at a spot in the middle of my thigh. I

rocked my wrist slowly. How easy it was to stick an orange, how difficult to jab my skin. I gathered up my courage and plunged it forward—but then stopped at the point of impact and eased it slowly, painfully downward. There is something about self-injection that makes one pause and go slowly, even though it is better to plunge right in.

The skin caved in because of my hesitation, until the flesh finally gave way and the needle slipped in. I had to run my hand along the syringe to get to the plunger. It would not give, and I began to fear that the needle would stay in my leg forever. Finally the insulin began to flow, raising a bump to the side of the injection point.

My skin puckered as I pulled the needle out, then snapped back when the needle was removed. I rubbed an alcohol swab over the point of injection. My leg began to hurt, and the ache did not leave that day. I knew I should not have gone so slowly.

When the nurse left I cried again, perhaps from the realization that I would have to do this every day for the rest of my life. I didn't know then that it would become a twice-daily ritual. I don't think it was the needle that bothered me so much as the fact that I could not live without the liquid in that bottle, that my life depended on it. It was a frightening and awesome prospect. To this day I still hesitate before taking an injection.

The doctor said I could go home the next day, and I was happy again at last. I thought everything would get back to normal once I was home.

It was just the beginning.

2

Normal?

MAY WAS WARMING into June when I came home from the hospital in 1964. I spent a great deal of time in the backyard, idly scraping my feet against the flagstone patio, watching the trim rows of bushes greening into new life. My parents had let me stay home because I was afraid to return to school, afraid that the other kids would notice a change in me.

I was gripped by the fear that I would wear my disease like a poster, that my classmates would be able to see the internal changes and mark me forever as different. Silly in retrospect, perhaps, but why do so few doctors bother to deal with this kind of problem?

Being branded by his peers is a frightening prospect for the diabetic child. It hardly matters that the fear is groundless. A child does not operate with logic: belief is everything. Whatever illusions the diabetic child creates *make* him different. These are the roots of psychological trauma, and from them come a plethora of reactions that lead to potentially dangerous health practices for the diabetic. It is the psychological factors that set off many of the physical complications of diabetes.

Diabetes is perhaps the only chronic disease in which the burden of responsibility lies almost totally with the patient. The goal is to attain a relatively stable blood-sugar level, but the process of life complicates the struggle. Attitudes—fears, doubts—affect the fragile balance. The child has an identity, a self-image, to form, and the juvenile diabetic cannot separate his disease from the growing process, because he lives with it every day. This fusion of mind and body is never easy to live with.

The doctor and my parents sat me down and tried to explain the concept of limitations, of control. If I followed all the rules, they said, I could lead a normal life. At ten, I did not understand how a life could be normal with those rules. Needles were not normal. Sticking to a diet was not normal. And what was the connection between a candy bar and the milky fluid in the syringe?

But I took the needle every day. I tested my urine every day, knowing only, as I dropped the pill into the test tube filled with urine, that an orange color was bad. I had no idea that what orange indicated was a high level of sugar spilling into the urine —another connection missing.

My single most persistent feeling then was of separation: *Other children do not take a needle. I cannot eat the same foods they do. I do not feel the same as I did before. I am different.* How easily resentment, struggle, and rebellion are created.

I cried my way into staying home from school for a week, but my mother, an intelligent woman blessed with kindness and good sense, knew that a week was enough; the spell of my grim little world had to be broken.

The usual routine in the morning: urine test, insulin injection; the feeling that this would never end, the realization that every morning for the rest of my life I would perform this ritual. But on this particular morning the dread was intense. I was going to school; my classmates would know I was different.

They will see through me, I thought. My hands began to shake. The back of my head itched. And I prayed to God to heal me. It was a simple matter of going to school—but it felt like a trip to the grave.

At school I sat at the polished wood desk, my head down, my eyes on the childish graffiti etched in the wood. I could not look the other kids in the face, could only shoot quick glances at the blackboard at the front of the room. Was everyone staring, or was my shame a product of my imagination?

Doctors often soothe the diabetic by saying that people have no way of knowing he has the disease. Comforting to an adult, perhaps, but to a child, surface appearance means nothing. I believed that my classmates could see through me. The damage done me was not inflicted by others, but came from within myself: I created the shame that damaged my identity. And of course, someone came along to reinforce my fears.

I don't remember his name, but I can never forget everything else about him. His frame was squat, his arms and legs short. His eyes were green, pushed to slits by the softness of his cheeks. His hair was red and curly, tight against the skull.

He walked over to me during recess. I was standing alone on the rim of the schoolyard, kicking stones against the fence, when I saw him coming. He stood a few feet away from me, a wide smile splitting his face. "Teacher told us you were in the hospital," he said.

My breathing got short. I did not answer. He knows, I thought, he knows.

"She told us what it was," he said.

I wanted to run, to push him aside and find a place where no one could see, no one would know.

"She said you were real sick and we had to be nice to you when you came back," he said. "You don't look so sick to me."

I didn't realize that he couldn't see the illness.

"She explained about diabetes; she said that's what you got." I met his eyes for a moment. "I never heard about that diabetes before, so I asked my mother. She said it was catching and to stay away from you or I'd get it, too."

So that was why he was keeping his distance. I was so terror-stricken that I could not reply.

"Why'd you come back to school?" he asked. "You want to make us all sick? You better stay away from *me.* "

He turned and walked off—and I never told a soul about the incident.

When I later learned that I could not spread the disease, I didn't feel much comforted. What other children thought of me was more important at that stage of my life than the actual truth. I felt set apart from my own small society. I was deeply, everlastingly lonely—and strongly resentful at having no control over the situation.

There was a pressure from within, straining outward to every cell of my body. It began as a tightness in my stomach and chest, and grew until every part of my frame was shaking. There was no way to control the spasms. Perspiration coated me from the back of my neck to the soles of my feet. And all the while there was the sense of a coming explosion, a feeling that my body would be ripped to shreds. The nervous system no longer paid attention to the brain. My heart pounded out of control, and I sucked in air spastically. Objects spun before my eyes. Concentration was impossible, and I began a slow drifting from reality. There had never been anything in the world like this. Fatigue spread through my body. I felt anger—senseless, un-controlled—and thought I was going mad.

I called my mother and told her something was happening to me. She recognized the signs and quickly gave me a candy bar to eat. I soon began to feel better.

This was my first insulin reaction, a process that can be frighteningly swift. It happens when the blood-sugar level falls too low, when a diabetic on insulin burns up sugar naturally, with exercise or overexertion. In my case, insulin reactions have always been fast and severe.

The one organ in the human body that needs sugar all the time is the brain. If blood sugar falls below a certain level, brain cells simply stop functioning. But that marvelous computer within the skull sends out a warning signal when the level becomes dangerous. The message runs along the sympathetic nervous system, which in turn strikes out at the body. These become the symptoms of the insulin reaction: the brain is telling the body it needs sugar.

Without insulin, there can be no life for the juvenile diabetic; yet insulin is the cause of this horrific reaction. That first time it happened to me, it was like being possessed, like stepping out of my body and watching it perform.

Ingestion of sugar can take care of the physical reaction, but it does nothing to soothe the mind. From that day on I lived in fear of insulin shock, in fear of my own body. All ideas of "normal" vanished in the wake of that single event.

I felt rejected by my body as well as by my friends, and I retreated from everyone. I was too afraid and confused to talk over my feelings of fear and resentment with either my parents or the doctor. Withdrawal is the worst possible reaction for the diabetic child; it is also, I believe, the most common.

Truth fosters acceptance. A child needs to know that an insulin reaction, though it comes, will go away. He must also realize that it will come back, but that he can fight it, that someone will be there to help him fight. If he cowers silently, too long by himself, he may actually rebel against help when he needs it.

It was a life of rules, and I began to hate them. Forbidden fruit: how delicious something looks when you are told you can't have it; how tempting to sneak a bite when no one is watching.

Before turning diabetic I did not have much of a sweet tooth, but afterward I became insatiable. It was the classic pattern of rebellion for the diabetic child. This early rebellion can, unfortunately, set the pattern for future complications more severe than a boy of ten could imagine. Kidneys and circulatory systems do not readily heal.

The needle is a force that rules a diabetic's life: he cannot live without insulin. And he is reminded every day of his life of this fact. The body becomes hostage to a vial of insulin, a very real form of confinement.

One might argue that food and water also confine mankind, and that diabetics should view insulin in this way. That sounds logical, but few diabetics would consider the argument fair: food and water can be skipped or delayed—and who stays constantly aware of the crucial role nutrition plays in our survival?

The swift and violent nature of the diabetic's physical reactions makes his sense of confinement intense. And the needle fosters rebellion. Because there is no way to fight the taking of insulin, the child fights in other ways.

Tell him he can't eat chocolates, that it's dangerous for him to drink Cokes. These forbidden pleasures then take on an irresistible lure.

I ate chocolates. I drank Cokes. I also skipped meals—to spite myself, to test my body. And, of course, I made life hell for my parents.

How, then, should a diabetic child be dealt with? It is the parents' task to watch over and guide him, and yet parental concern is such a painful reminder of the diabetic's condition that the concern in itself can give rise to resentment.

In most cases, the resentment dissipates as the child matures, but I think it is important in the early stages to ease up on pep talks about "normalcy," at best a faulty concept. We are all individuals, and the diabetic child should be approached with his singularity in mind. If he learns compassion from the experience of his pain, his own sense of humanity will be enriched. If he learns patience from the frustration of his position, he has taken another big step toward maturity. And if someone listens to his fears and shows him understanding, he may himself become blessed with concern for others.

Hope and faith are strong human tonics, the elixir of dreams and aspirations. Belief, which gives us the strength to go on in moments of crisis, can brighten a dark hour. But when dreams are destroyed, they become a terrible burden to the psyche.

I dreamed for nothing less than a miracle—and after a few weeks the miracle seemed to be happening. Insulin reactions became regular events, so the doctor kept lowering my dosage: I got down to the minimal two units a day. How I prayed for the two units to drop to zero—it would mean the difference

between two worlds, two people, signaling a return to the old
world of comfort and serenity.

Every night the repetitious prayer: Please, Jesus, make it go
away, make me normal. I have tried to be good, watch over me
and make me well. You healed the sick and turned water into
wine. Turn my body into what it was. Heal me, Jesus, please
heal me.

And then the answer came.

The doctor said to stop taking insulin. He said this was often
possible after a few weeks of treatment, but that I should not
expect to be healed. But results make a strong impression: I was
off insulin, I would stay off. For a week I thought the world was
wonderful again—maybe. Always in the back of my mind was
the fear that the reaper would return.

I later learned that there are rare instances of spontaneous
remission, but mine was not such a case. The diabetes returned
after seven days, and with it, a more intense feeling of abandon-
ment and betrayal—God had played a cruel trick on me. At ten,
I lost all faith and gave up on the world.

By not taking care of myself, I had once thought I was getting
back at forces I could not control, but now I saw that there was
nothing, and no one else, to fight. So I waged a one-man cam-
paign of anger on the battlefield of the self. There could be only
one loser.

3

Images of Death

I AM SCARED all the time. I am afraid of darkness and shadows. I live in dread of the physical reactions that rock my body in the middle of the night, of the pain centered in my lower back and of the imaginary picture of my kidneys dissolving and passing through my urine. I tremble at the thought of an amputated foot—blood pouring onto the operating table, and later the long, thick scar of a stump. But it is the grim, eternal night of darkness that I fear the most—the possibility that one day blindness will descend and I will never see light again. I am afraid today, and every day.

These fears, stemming from the reality of diabetes, impose crippling restrictions on the movement of a life and construct barriers in the mind that could lead to madness: the madness of confinement, alienation, loneliness; a mind in torment, a consciousness weighed down by the possibility of physical pain. I am human and I am afraid. I feel a terrible sense of loss and regret when thinking of the past, cannot separate moments of contentment and joy from the constant fear of the disease. Diabetes hangs over my entire past, staining all recollections, because as a child what I saw in my disease was the mystery of blackness within. And what came from within I interpreted as a product of the self. The conclusion: I myself am the blackness.

I remember, from the time I was ten, being afraid of the dark. It seems to me now a symbol of that time in my life, a period of mystery filled with pain and secret obsessions. To move away from parents and friends was instinctive. But the night revealed the true nature of isolation, when there is no distraction from oneself, when every reaction of the body seems more acute. The night turned into a battlefield of mind and body.

At night, if I thought of all the simple pleasures that a child takes for granted, I also thought of how quickly such comforts could be taken away—as quickly as the disease had snatched my health and my peace. Every memory became tinged with sadness, permeated with a sense of loss.

I remember my grandfather. He was small but powerfully built, with a full head of white hair and fingers that were gnarled, thick, stained yellow by tobacco. I remember sitting with him on the gray stoop as he tried to teach me how to roll his cigarettes. He would laugh and rub my head as the paper and tobacco were destroyed by my hands. He would explain again the proper method, step by step, as he rolled a perfect tube. He would smoke it down until it burned his fingers.

Grandpa was not supposed to smoke. Grandpa was a diabetic.

He got the disease late in life and was told he would just have to watch his diet. Maturity-onset diabetes probably has some foundation in heredity, but it is probably also a result of diet.

In any case, it is a fact that maturity-onset diabetics have a high percentage of diabetic relatives.

He was not a "good" diabetic and seemed unable to develop any discipline about what he ate. Ignorance was not the problem; though he had not had much schooling, he was blessed with a fine intelligence. He listened to the radio for hours at a time, and commented on every subject imaginable. His language was a charming mixture of Italian and English, but no one ever had trouble understanding him.

I believe he chose to ignore the disease because the small habits of a lifetime are a comfort in later years. In saying this, I do not mean to recommend his behavior. It is simply that I understand his motives. Toward the end he suffered, and his life span was certainly greatly reduced because he didn't follow the proper diet.

It is curious that we never spoke of the disease we had in common. I have never, in fact, discussed diabetes with any others in my family who have the disease. Grandpa and I had a closeness and affection that went beyond words. We sat on the stoop and talked about the formations of stars in the sky, the time he spent in a prison camp in World War I, of his twin brother who had lived in Argentina and died at an early age. Later, I realized that his brother had probably also been diabetic and hadn't received proper medical attention.

So he would not change his ways, this marvelous old man whom I loved so dearly and still miss so much. At home, in Brooklyn, he pressed grapes in the basement for his supply of wine; he would not give up his vino. It seemed to me, even then, more than a matter of just giving up the pleasure of alcohol. It was the whole process of making the product that was dear to him, that must have been such a comfort in a mechanized world moving by too fast.

If he lived a shorter life, he lived it well. But I still feel a mixture of terror and pain when I think of the day he sat drinking beer in the kitchen, can still hear the sound of the glass shattering and see his head falling forward. He had a stroke that summer day, an occurrence often related to diabetes of some duration. They carried him to the sofa, and I can see him smiling as he came to. In his pain, he smiled, and I wanted to tell him how much I loved him and what a courageous man he was. How I wanted to be like him—to wake up smiling and ignore the fear and pain. From that day until he died, he lived with the pain, but always smiled. He suffered from arteriosclerosis and heart disease; the diabetes had traveled through his blood vessels and exacted an awesome toll. And still, in the hospital, I saw him smoking.

He lingered on for about two years, but his gait had become slow and painful, and his entire body deteriorated. In its final phase, diabetes becomes a blanket disease, and complications spread to every part of the body: the eyes, the extremities, the circulatory system, the kidneys, liver, heart, brain.

His death was a direct result of diabetes. If his kidneys refused to function, it was because of diabetes; if his heart gave in, it stopped because the sugar corroded his system.

I gazed at his face, so peaceful in death, and felt an odd sense of betrayal. He was gone, and I would miss the charm of his ways, his tenderness, the strength of his presence. But he had left me, and though we had never talked of diabetes, that bond between us had been a source of comfort. Now that he was dead, I made the obvious connection: Grandpa was a diabetic; Grandpa had died; I am a diabetic . . .

He was buried on a hot summer Sunday, and only one detail remains vivid in my mind. We stood at the grave site and I tried to hold back my tears, to act brave. Once the words were said, the casket was lowered into the ground, and one by one we filed past the grave. When I reached the open pit I paused, a blood-red, long-stemmed rose in my hand. I let go of the stem and watched the flower drop into the vastness of the earth. And it struck me that this gesture was so small and insignificant, yet all I could now ever do for a man I had loved intensely.

I turned from the grave and walked back to the car, and it was then that the tears came in waves, my body uncontrolled and shaking. For the rest of the afternoon I cried: at the mystery of pain and loss, the insignificance of dreams in the face of reality, the confinement of body, the matters out of human control. I cried at the loss of hope and faith. And I cried because I was alone.

The diabetic mind is one that interprets many events and ideas through their connection with the disease. There is often no logic to this habit of thought, but it works nonetheless on the personality.

I was going to a Catholic school the year I became a diabetic. On the first Friday of every month a mass was attended by all the students. The nuns lined us in neat rows on the hardwood pews. And we pushed back the kneelers and held our backs erect.

On the first mass after my return from the hospital, I was torn with doubt about the Creator. I had been made sick; the sickness had abandoned my body for a week, and then like some cruel joke had returned. I knew there was only one force in the universe that could control such matters. I was sitting in His house.

The high, arched ceiling reached toward Heaven, and the stained-glass panels threw colored shadows along the length of the congregation. A red carpet formed a long trail down the

center aisle, leading up the marble steps to the altar and taber-
nacle, which contained the golden chalice. A silver gate separated God's realm from His servants. Thick white candles
formed a triangle: small ones at the ends, encased in metal
brackets rising in perfect formation toward the center. A tribute
to God.

I will never forget those candles: they came to haunt my
dreams, to give rise to horror in the middle of the night.

For the faithful, the candles represent the power of light, the
illumination of the spirit. We see in this light goodness, and
protection; we strive for its brilliance by communion with the
Creator. I did not think it ironic then that this symbol of light
takes the form of fire, that light can become a force of destruction.

The voice of the priest boomed through the vastness of the
church, telling us that preparation for the Eucharist was the
very focus of our lives, a gift so powerful that we could never
be worthy of it. But God in His wisdom had allowed us sinners
to partake of His body and blood, and such a gift should not
be declined.

The altar boys, in ornate cassock and surplice, moved in
circles around the priest during the ritual of Consecration.
Their robes gave them authority in the service of the Lord.
Their movements were quick and stiff as they went to the side
of the priest. At the moment of Consecration, one altar boy
swept to the side to ring the bells, his silk-trimmed cassock
trailing behind him.

Over the years, I have replayed the same scene thousands of
times: The spin of the boy's form as he reaches for the bells. The
draft from his swirling cassock. The candle. Flame flickers, dies
for a moment. Silk. He ignites. The silk trim explodes, and he
is devoured by flame.

Dear God, he is burning to death.

He screamed, a fireball dancing around the altar. The house of God was filled with the smell of burning flesh. We sat, silent and paralyzed. A nun screamed. The priest ran to the flaming boy, caught him and threw him to the floor. He rolled the flames in the red carpet that ran the length of the church. Smoke poured from the open ends of the rolled carpet. The priest cradled the boy in his arms and carried him out of the church.

We were told to pray for the safety of the altar boy, and we sat for what seemed like hours. When the priest returned, he moved to the lectern with tears in his eyes. His voice cracked through the speakers, exploding the stunned silence of the congregation. The boy was dead—he had burned to death. He told us we would continue the mass to pray for the boy's soul.

It was the proper thing to do, but I just wanted to leave. I gagged when the wafer touched my tongue, became sick with the odor in the church. This symbol of life and goodness was tinged with the smell of death, and I could not separate the two. My relationship with God was confused enough before, but now there was the smell of burning flesh in His house. Death was swift; even in the house of God, death was swift and merciless.

Juvenile diabetes imposes a strain on any family. Parents become guardians, the keepers of order and balance. The diabetic's special needs often pose problems for the other children, who may feel ignored and resentful. Family life can become a powder keg. I have a great deal of respect for my brothers and sister because they never resented my disease, my personal problems, or my relations with our parents. The opposite was true: at times their own concern bordered on overprotection.

There are six members of the family, and I often had five parents.

My brother Ralph is eighteen months older than I. We were constant childhood companions—and more, we were good friends. My memories of our early years are filled with joy. But in a spirit of love and respect I feel it is time to register one complaint to him: Did you have to take me to that movie, you bastard?

You know now what I'm talking about. But I suppose you couldn't have known then the kind of terror and dread it inspired in me on that cool Sunday as we sat in the theater eating popcorn. I wanted to leave even before the opening credits had finished rolling, but you must have thought I was joking. It was that first diabetic year, and I was seeing pain and death in every dark chamber of my imagination. What a morbid child I was —four feet tall and one foot already in the grave.

The film opens on the damp, dark streets of London. It is night in the city, and the cobblestones gleam with a thin film of moisture. Hansom cabs throw long, sinister shadows across the pavement, and the sound of hoofbeats mingles with the background music. The shadow of a man plays across the screen.

The camera pans along the length of the shadow, concentrating on the man's feet as he moves slowly through the city. The sound of footsteps assaults the ears as the shadow enters a tunnel. Something moves in the dark area to the right. Laughter. Then moans. The camera moves closer: a seedy man presses close to a young whore, trapping her in a doorway.

The shadow pauses; moves on.

Farther down the street, another young whore leans against the railing of a stoop. She paints her lips and brushes back her curls as she looks in the direction of the footsteps. A smile breaks the line of her full, red lips. The footsteps become louder, until the head of the shadow covers her face. She lifts her head and her welcoming smile turns into terror, her mouth stretching open to scream.

A knife, the biggest knife I have ever seen, flashes across the width of the screen in living color, the light from a gas streetlamp reflecting off the blade. The blade enters the right side of the whore's neck and makes a clean exit on the left. Blood spurts down her throat and into her golden curls. Her eyes and mouth remain open. A black-gloved hand lets go of the knife, but it remains impaled in the woman's neck. The blood pours down her dress, Hollywood blood that just doesn't stop running.

The camera remained fixed on the scene as the credits and title began to fill the screen. I should have left then, because the opening was tame compared with the rest of the picture: Jack the Ripper, with Sherlock Holmes on his trail, slit throats, severed heads and limbs, mutilated bodies—all of it close up and bloody beyond belief.

I can laugh about it now, but I didn't sleep that Sunday night after the movie, and it was years before I could get all that blood out of my mind. Sherlock Holmes caught his man, but he did not corner death itself. And death came to diabetics . . .

My cousin Frankie was a diabetic, and between us there was that same silent bond I had had with my grandfather. We never talked about the disease. I knew nothing about Frankie's insulin dose or his diet, and it never crossed either of our minds to ask; it was enough just to know we were both diabetics. We would run together through the woods in back of the house, throw rocks in the stream, and laugh with delight when a fish jumped in the water.

Frankie was my junior by three years, but he is no longer alive. He died when he was nine.

At the time, I was not told what he died of, nor was I taken to the funeral. I learned later that his death was related to diabetes, but I think the effect on me would not have been any different if he had been hit by a car. By then diabetes and my fear of death were so intertwined that I had come to think that diabetes *meant* death.

There would have been no way to convince me that the deaths of my grandfather and my cousin were not in some way connected to my own fate. There was no way I would have believed that those bloody prostitutes littering the streets of London would rise and walk again. Burdened with fears, my mind refused to reason. If the wind blew the smoke from a neighbor's fireplace toward us, I thought our house was burning down.

The fears grew, until, at the age of thirteen, I could not sleep on Sunday nights. It made no sense, but it was only Sunday night. On the seventh day the Creator rested; on the seventh day I could not sleep. Consumed by anxiety, I was terrified that if I went to sleep I would die. Every creak in the house was an imagined killer stalking dark corners.

I began to check all the doors and windows before I went to bed. At times this procedure would take more than an hour. I placed my hand over the gas pilot on the stove, waiting until the heat transferred to my fingers. I had visions of the house exploding in a fireball.

In time, I worked my way through the fears. I believe now that their source was a combination of events: my grandfather's death, the fire in the church (which I apparently associated with Sunday, making an obvious connection, although it actually happened on a Friday), the movie on a Sunday afternoon.

Years later, I learned that my cousin Frankie had died on a Sunday night.

4

Invalid

IT WAS THE FIRST—and last—theft I have ever committed. It was probably the worst thing I could have stolen at the age of thirteen, not because the caper would lead me to a life of crime, but because my loot was poison, and I could have killed myself with it. The crime was premeditated; my stupidity was astounding. There were no cautions printed on the bottle, no skull and crossbones on the label, yet I knew it was poison for me.

It happened because I was feeling like an invalid. The diabetic, more than anyone around him, *makes himself* feel this way. The young diabetic is afraid of his disorder, and he tends to resent guidance and care because they are reminders of the fears he is trying to suppress. A common reaction is to rebel against all forms of control—behavior that can pose tremendous problems during adolescence.

Though there are no firm statistics, a doctor once told me that the suicide rate for diabetics is much higher than the norm for the general population. But I was not suffering from suicidal tendencies, just stupidity. I was thirteen years old and trying to fit in, afraid of being rejected by my peers.

After a week of plotting, I stole a bottle of Dewar's Scotch from my father's stock in the basement. I had never even tasted liquor, but my sole intention was to get dead drunk.

My accomplice in crime was a boy named Donald, older by a year and reputedly wise in the ways of the world. He was short and lean, and had a long, narrow face with a bulbous nose. Donald was an absolute dictionary of obscene terms, and commanded the respect of all the neighborhood teenagers. That mouth—how loud and lewd that mouth was! His status was also heightened because he had found a stack of his father's old *Playboy*s in the basement, and the puberty crowd would sit and gawk at them on the damp concrete floor on rainy days.

I remember that Donald once called me a hard-on in front of my father. I had never heard the term, but my father was upset and took me upstairs for a man-to-man session. He said it was a bad word, and I asked him what it meant. He told me it was when your penis became hard. I imagined a petrified or rotting tree, and for a few years afterward I was afraid of the hard-on disease—if the penis got hard it would fall off.

Well, I was plainly out of Donald's league. He made fun of me because I had never been drunk. He called me a mama's boy, a pussycat. He knew I was a diabetic, but he had no idea of what having the disease meant. If I got a bottle, he said, he would show me how to drink.

The bottles were kept in the cedar closet in the basement, along with clothes and other things. The closet was always kept locked. My mother gave us the key when she wanted us to fetch something. On one such trip I left the door unlocked intentionally. My mother asked if I had shut it; I answered "Yes," and handed her the key.

I reported to Donald that I could get the bottle any time, and he said we would get drunk on Sunday. (Again an event on *Sunday* was to play a crucial role in my life.) That Sunday we went to a confirmation party for one of my cousins. It was getting late and I was supposed to meet Donald at five. I can't remember the excuses I made, but I kept badgering my father, telling him I wanted to go home. He finally gave in, and my uncle Tom drove me home. I wished later he had known what was on my mind.

Out of habit, I checked all the doors and windows in the house, then crept into the basement. My parents are not drinkers, but my father always kept the basement well stocked for family gatherings and guests. Cases were stacked on the floor of the closet. I opened a box at random, my hands shaking with excitement, and took out a bottle of Dewar's.

It was a warm May evening, and I walked to Donald's house, the bottle tucked under my arm. I held it behind my back as I rang the doorbell. I didn't ever remember his mother answering the door, so I was not afraid of discovery.

Donald appeared. He looked me over and broke into a smile. "Do you have it?"

I spat on the ground to convey the absurdity of the question, thinking that I must look very cool and collected. I spread my legs and rocked on the balls of my feet. "What do you think?" I said. "I told you I could get it."

I pulled the bottle from behind my back. He took it in his hands, turned it slowly, made a long inspection of the label. "Good stuff," he said. "And it's a whole quart; bigger than the usual. We can really get plastered." Then, probably because I looked as proud of myself as I felt, Donald had to assert his superiority. "But this shit might be more than *you* can take."

I had to find a way to save face. "You kidding?" I said. "Reason I picked the De-war's was because I really want to get bombed."

"Do-ers, you schmuck, Do-ers. Baby. Guess I'll have to show you how."

I decided I was in the care of a master, so I let him take charge. He had found the perfect spot, a golf course that bordered a road in back of our houses and was surrounded by thick woods. Donald held the bottle as we walked through the brush. We came to a small clearing with a dead tree trunk on the ground. Cigarette butts were littered around the tree. This was the neighborhood meeting place for illicit teenage activities.

Donald sat on the trunk and opened the bottle. "Drink it right down," he said. "That's all there is to it." He took a short swig and, trying not to gag, passed it over.

I hesitated, wondering how you actually got drunk; Donald certainly didn't look drunk. I took a gulp and the taste was so sickening that I spat it out.

"You have to hold it down if you want to get drunk," he said, and took another short swig.

I grabbed the bottle and tilted my head far back, forcing the Scotch down my throat. My stomach was instantly repelled, but I kept the liquor down by sheer force of will. I glanced at Donald, puzzled. "I'm not drunk," I said. "It isn't working."

He laughed. "Idiot," he said. "You have to drink a lot more than that to get drunk—you have to put away at least half the bottle, and pretty fast, at that."

He was the expert, I the fool. I took his advice and downed half a quart in less than ten minutes. Donald laughed as he watched, but he did not try to take the bottle from me. I doubt if he drank very much at all that night.

I complained again: "It ain't working," I said. "The crap doesn't work."

"Have a little more," he said.

My determination was strong, but my stomach would take no more. Since that day I have always found the taste and smell of Scotch sickening. "We'd better try another night," I said. "I don't think it's going to work."

A short time later it started working.

I felt a warm tingle in my head that soon spread to every part of my body. My eyes began to go out of focus. I stared at Donald's nose, and for some reason thought its bulk extremely funny. I rolled on the ground and laughed uncontrollably.

"It's starting to work," he said.

I didn't answer. I stood up and started taking off all my clothes. I danced an elaborate striptease, bumping my hips against the trees.

Donald laughed. "What d'ya think you're doin'?" he asked. "Put your clothes back on."

I began to dance a wild jig, bare-assed naked in the woods. My arms were heavy and my breathing short.

"I'm a bear!" I yelled. "I'm a dancing bear!" My body was rocked by convulsive laughter, and I arched backward.

With that I fell into a stream.

My arms pumped wildly in the water. Mud splattered my face and chest. I began to scream. "Something's biting my ass! It's going to bite it off!" I couldn't get out of the water. "Save me," I screamed. "Save me."

He pulled me out of the water and tried to dry my body with leaves. My head began to spin when I closed my eyes. I passed out for a time, then woke to a face-slapping. The night was now pitch-black and silent.

Then the stomach convulsions came in waves, and the vomit

poured from my mouth and nose. My stomach burned and my lungs gasped for breath.

"I knew you couldn't take it," said Donald.

I passed out again.

Donald somehow managed to dress me. I have no recollection of the trip home except for one small detail: I remember falling in the gutter and scraping my hand.

Donald later told me that I threw up on at least six of the neat lawns in the neighborhood during the journey home. I also reputedly urinated on a fire hydrant and attempted to rape a tree.

I have no recollection of entering the house or preparing for bed. I do remember my relief when I found the house empty. I somehow managed to change my clothes and get into the bed.

I passed out again.

The next thing I remember is my mother screaming that I was drunk and trying to lift me from the bed. By this time my body was trembling and was covered with a film of sweat. When I stood up I began to puke again, and my mother led me to the bathroom.

I am alive today because my mother knew what was taking place inside my body.

Alcohol raises the blood sugar considerably when consumed in large amounts—half a bottle of Scotch, for instance. The real danger, however, is that after a certain length of time the sugar takes a quick plunge. For the diabetic on insulin, this effect poses the danger of insulin reaction.

I needed sugar in my body. Simple. But in my state I couldn't hold anything down. The insulin reaction was becoming serious, and I was on the verge of losing consciousness.

We spent most of the night in the bathroom, my mother and I. With patience bordering on sainthood she fed me apples, one after the other. As soon as I took a few bites, I would promptly throw up.

And so we passed the night.

She fed me an apple.

I threw up.

Another apple.

I retched some more.

Another apple.

I passed out.

She slapped me awake.

Another apple.

Finally I had ingested enough sugar to be out of danger.

Left on my own, I would most likely have died in my sleep. All because I wanted to fit in, because of foolish childhood notions of normalcy and an inner voice telling me to rebel against the label "invalid."

It didn't work. It never does. If I learned a lesson that night, it was that I need never fear becoming an alcoholic. I would be dead long before I could ever reach that stage.

5

A Healing Summer

THE DISMAL FAILURE of my experiment with alcohol rein-
forced the idea that in my whole being I was different from the
people around me. My adolescent attempt at social acceptance
only strengthened the reality that I could not act like others,
and this realization deepened my feelings of resentment and
injustice.

So once again I experienced that deep sense of confinement
that comes with the realization that the body is out of control.
I prepared the insulin injection every morning, not in the spirit
of thanksgiving, but resenting the fact that my life was controlled by the substance in the vial. Insulin is extracted from
pork and beef, and the longer-acting suspensions work by the
addition of various substances, including zinc, protein from
beef blood, and even the sperm of rainbow trout. It is humbling
for a diabetic to learn how he is kept alive.

That kind of total dependence overpowers the striving of the adolescent for identity. Diabetes, it seemed to me, interfered with *everything*—and produced an early obsession with death.

So I was, at the age of fifteen, a morbid boy who sat in his room reading books and writing odes to the Angel of Death. Fear makes us shut out the world, and the strongest image of my adolescence was closing the door of my own dark chamber, shutting out all the sounds and movements of life.

It is ironic that the cure was so simple, something that lifted the tremendous weight of years: talking about it. The problem was that it was the last thing in the world I wanted to do; I tried, in fact, to avoid all human contact. I created my own hell for many years.

My parents saw me become depressed and withdrawn, and were saddened, I realize now, by the loss of their once vibrant child. They tried to help, asked often what was bothering me. Their pain may have been greater than my own. Parents often suffer more than an afflicted child, especially when the disease is believed to be hereditary. Mine were, I think, often as confused as I, and to add to their burden, I would never say what was on my mind. I sat in my room and brooded, wept at the most insignificant of probings, inclined easily toward anger and rage.

What was I raging against? Seeing others function in ways I never could; foolishly believing that they could never understand the intense pain I was suffering. Not the outward pain of the needle or a nervous sytem out of control, but rather the inner torment of the fear of death. Fear born of specifics: a fire in church, a Sunday movie, the death of two relatives . . .

So I cut everyone off and refused to talk with members of my family, friends, teachers. The house was a battleground for my frustrations, and no matter how hard my family tried to comfort me, I would snap at them and close them off. There was nothing they could really do. Communication was impossible because of my attitude; it was also my strongest need.

I acted the same way with my doctor, who probably understood my reaction but couldn't help either. I think the only time I opened my mouth was when he checked my throat. Dr. Reese, to whom I was referred by the doctor who diagnosed my condition, is a diabetic specialist—and the finest, most understanding doctor who has ever treated me. I cannot overstress the importance of a concerned physician. Poor attitudes go back to the onset of diabetes; the doctor is the one to attach a name to the frightening, disorienting symptoms, and the way he handles this traumatic moment can have long-lasting effects on the diabetic.

Today, I have no quarrel with the medical profession. I judge doctors as individuals; like the rest of us, they can be greedy, unconcerned, or even ignorant. The patient retains the tremendous responsibility of turning over the care of his body, not to a god, but to someone who is just another human being. I spell this out because I once placed blind faith in doctors. As a result, I have more than once come close to losing my life.

So how does a juvenile diabetic break out of such a self-destructive mold? I have always felt comforted in the presence of another diabetic, but I find that diabetics rarely compare notes about their emotions. For a fifteen-year-old, the need to talk is crucial. If the silence goes on for very long, the burden can become too great. The mind can bend, but at some point it will snap from the weight. And the diabetic's state of mind affects control of the disease.

I was saved that summer in part by physical work. I got a job in the kitchen of a summer day camp, and found comfort and pleasure in sheer physical exertion. I would swing a mop brutally from side to side along the endless gray floor. I would stack garbage cans high and then carry them outside. I washed a thousand forks and knives a day, carried endless cartons of milk that were covered with huge blocks of ice. We cooked food in eight large ovens, sweated from the heat as we boiled fifty-gallon vats of tomato sauce. I forgot myself when working, forgot the pain, the fear, the feelings of rejection.

I was having insulin reactions every day from all this exertion, but I would quickly swallow sweets so I could hurry back to work. I was too busy to let my dangerous imagination run wild; I had found another outlet for all the frustration. I felt a deep sense of satisfaction when the campers would come teeming into the dining room, twelve hundred strong, rushing to eat what I had helped prepare. I was valuable, in spite of my disease. I was beginning to see life, not death in the movements of the world. And that simple change in thinking covered a distance so vast it seemed almost miraculous.

How I loved that work, how good it felt to sweat from physical exertion rather than the nervous tremblings of an insulin reaction. Slowly the job itself broke down many of the barriers in my mind, began giving me a good image of myself.

There were several other boys in the kitchen crew, and after we finished working we would roam the grounds, talk, and play games. Most of us became friends. We spent a lot of our time devising shortcuts for our work.

One day I had the brilliant idea of mopping the floor with a mixture of ammonia and bleach. I reasoned that ammonia cut grease, and bleach whitened. I was delighted when the mixture started smoking, but then I almost passed out: I didn't know the mixture was poisonous.

Freddy dragged me out of the kitchen.

I met him on the first day of camp—a handsome, trim boy with an eagle beak. He came right over and started talking. I thought him funny, wise, and literate for a boy my own age. He spoke softly and listened well.

We became a team, Freddy and I, in search of an audience: he turned me into an extrovert. We laughed and joked, lounged in the storage basement, resting our heads on twenty-pound bags of rice, talking of the mysteries of sex and our dreams for the future. We lamented the fact that most of the women counselors were older than we. (They in turn teased us by saying it was a shame we were too young.) And so Freddy and I sat, two boasting fifteen-year-olds, lamenting the injustice of the fact that these girls would never know the pleasures of our bodies because of their closed minds. As silly as it may seem in retrospect, those sessions paved the way for a self-image that was slowly losing its preoccupation with diabetes.

I had taken a step toward restoring my mental health, but I was still not a "good" diabetic. One does not always learn by experience: I had sworn to myself at thirteen that I would never touch another drink, but Freddy and I would go into the basement several times a week and drink whatever we could get our hands on. My brother Ralph, who was in charge of the kitchen, would often find an excuse to run out to the store in the camp wagon, and would come back with bottles of wine and beer.

I had devised an elaborate system to keep the alcohol from interfering with my diabetes. Before beginning to drink, I would eat something sweet. As I drank, I could feel the sugar rising, because by this time my body was attuned to the changes taking place within. Then I would feel the sudden drop in my blood-sugar level, and at just the right time I would take large amounts of sugar into my system.

This was one way of staving off an insulin reaction, but such great fluctuations in sugar level do damage to the system, and I knew it. In addition, with all the drinking and the eating of sugar, my blood was bombarded for a long time afterward with a high excess of glucose. Instead of doing myself in quickly, I had begun a process of slow degeneration.

Why was I such an idiot? Why insist on damaging my body when I knew the potential dangers? The answer is just that it *felt* good to sit in that cool basement and talk with someone, a pleasure lost for so many years—a pleasure beyond description for a lonely teenager.

When I think of that summer I am bathed in feelings of warmth. It signaled the healing of wounds, the lifting of psychological burdens. I was learning to function in the real world, and though my disease was always present, the important thing was that I was learning to forget my fears for a time, even though I still dreaded the coming of night and darkness.

My reactions have always been excessive, and this period of my life, too, was marked by emotional highs and lows. I was often overexuberant, but any symbol or reminder of death was enough to bring me down with haunting depression: a crushed dog on the divider of a highway; the numbing exposure by the news media of the Vietnam War. I could not read the papers, was moved to tears by the cruelty and violence of the human race.

It was a hot, humid day in July. I was mopping one of the huge dining rooms. Sweat ran down my forehead and spilled into my eyes, and I had to sit down every few minutes to wipe my face. I removed my shirt and twisted it in my hands, watching a stream of perspiration fall to the floor. I was afraid of getting an insulin reaction, so I stopped for something cool and sweet to drink. The afternoon sun was beginning to fade, casting long shadows along the length of the dining room.

Freddy came in and sat on one of the long gray benches. He had finished his work and was wiping down his bare chest with a white towel. "Do you need any help?" he asked.

He knew I was a diabetic, but was the first person I ever met who did not seem mystified by the disease. It was not that he understood the ailment, it was just that he chose to ignore it and treat me like any other person. He did not ask endless questions.

My arms were trembling from the weight of the soaked mop. "I can use a hand," I said. "I just can't seem to get anything done today. I've never been this late before."

He went off for another mop and came back to help.

"Is something wrong?" he asked.

I stopped working and leaned on the mop. "I just feel tired today," I said. "I feel weak."

He stopped and leaned on his own mop, both of us in the same position, like matching bookends. "It must be the heat," he said. "It really gets to me sometimes."

We were both quiet for a long time, neither of us working, paralyzed over the mops. I was wondering if Freddy had ever been scared because of illness. And suddenly something gave me the courage to ask, "Have you ever felt really sick? I mean, were you ever really afraid that you might die?"

He looked up, twisting the mop handle, and his eyes told me I had found someone who would understand.

"When I was five, I had something wrong with my heart," he said. "It was missing beats, and I had to stay in bed for a long time. I couldn't go out and play with the other kids." He paused for what seemed like a long time. "I was afraid I was going to die, and I used to cry because I wasn't like the other kids. I thought I would spend the rest of my life in bed."

An enormous pressure was lifted from me at that moment, and everything I had been silent about for five years began to pour out. I told Freddy how much I hated the fact that I needed insulin to keep me alive, of my frustration at being dependent on the needle at a time in life when all my friends were so carefree. I talked about my fear of death, of how two close diabetic relatives had died, one slowly and painfully, and the other with frightening, cruel swiftness. I talked of how much I feared the reactions of my body, how during an insulin reaction everything went out of control and I seemed to be going mad. And I talked of God, of how he had left me to suffer, had even abandoned an altar boy in church. How I hated and feared all these things, how confused I was and tired of dealing with mysteries. I told him how removed I felt, how hard it was to discuss all these things, because I thought no one would understand or listen.

And he said something absolutely remarkable for a fifteen-year-old: "We're all afraid of things we can't control. It helps to talk, because that's really the only thing you *can* do."

The result of our talk was nothing less than a miracle. A healing of wounds, produced by simple human kindness, an understanding friend. A building of confidence until the mind becomes strong, turns from morbidity to a burning will to live and fight. It was a new attitude, a simple change of mind—and it is a crucial step in the development of a diabetic. To live with fear is damaging, but it is all too often the plight of the diabetic. To finally open up and talk is, I believe, literally life-saving.

There was a calming in my life, an easing of pressure that was essential at the time. I suspect that I might have gone mad were it not for the understanding Freddy offered me then.

This easing was a blessing, because later on I was engulfed by a second wave of fears: awareness of the future—indeed, the fear that there might not be a future.

When the diabetic becomes aware of the complications of his disease, this second wave hits with the force of a hurricane.

6

Freedom and Fear

AT THE AGE of seventeen I was about to leave home for the first time in my life. I had fought with my parents repeatedly over attending an out-of-town college. They were motivated by concern, and their logic was well founded: I did not have a very good track record when it came to caring for myself. In fact, I was almost always in a state of high blood sugar, feeling constantly weak, dry, and irritable. I thought I was getting away with something. The reality is that very few juvenile diabetics in poor control suffer immediately, but oh, what a price you pay later on.

My parents wanted me to stay at home because they did not believe I could survive if left on my own. That only made me resentful; I thought if I didn't break away, I would never escape that old label "invalid." When I think back to it now, I am deeply touched by my parents' concern. But at the time, I was trying very hard to convince myself that I could lead a normal life.

I felt I had to get away from the protection of home so that I could deal with the problems I had created. I needed to come to terms with diabetes in my own way, to deal with the doubts in my mind in solitude. It seemed too easy to stay at home and be pampered. I needed to see if I could function in the real world as a diabetic, to fall on my face as a test of strength. Would I be able to get up?

I was accepted at Boston University and told my parents I wanted to go there. They were against my going so far from New York, but my father agreed to fly up to Boston and look over the campus. I am not sure what changed his mind, but he was enchanted as we drove down Commonwealth Avenue. I think he finally realized that it might be best if I learned to handle life on my own.

In September I was about to embark on my great experiment. I was scared to death. I would have to form new routines; and habits play a large role in the life of a diabetic. I had always taken my needle in the same place and at the same time each day. What if I forgot to take it? What if I was alone and had an insulin reaction in the middle of the night? How would I find a doctor if I was very ill?

My father and brother packed the car while I said good-bye to my mother. She was crying as she gave last-minute instructions. She told me I could always come home. I knew she feared for my health.

It seemed like such a long drive. My father and brother talked in the front seat. I sat in the back, silent, my fear rising in direct proportion to the distance we had covered.

When we arrived in Boston my father took us out to dinner. Back at the dorm, we met my roommate and his family. His mother saw a package of needles on the bed and asked what they were. My father said I was a junkie. It took a while to calm her down and explain.

Originally, they were going to spend the night, but my father decided it might be better if they drove right home. I wanted them to stay, but did not say anything. I walked them to the car and watched them drive away. I was totally alone for the first time in my life, and I was frightened.

I did not sleep that night. I walked through the streets of Boston, gazing at statues; I sat on a bench in the Public Garden and began to cry. I circled the John Hancock tower and headed into the downtown district, swung back past the ornate brownstones of Beacon Hill, finally arriving back on campus.

I sat on a bench in front of the school chapel. Stray students would stop and talk, but I have no recollection of any of the people I met that night. I sat in the cool night air because I was afraid to go to sleep, afraid to be alone. I had wanted independence, but knew nothing of the responsibility that comes with it. At home, I could shut myself in my room, but in the back of my mind I always knew that if something went wrong, if I was ever in real physical danger, all I had to do was yell and someone would be at my side in minutes. No more.

I was struck now by the realization that I was alone in a city of strangers. I could fall in the street and be left there for days. I didn't know a single person in this city, could not turn to anyone in time of need. There was no one to remind me to take my insulin or eat at the proper time. In short, I had to learn to care for my own body. There was no one to do it for me.

I survived that first night. And the next. I was always amazed to find myself whole when I jumped out of bed in the morning, and as funny as it may seem, the simple fact of waking and functioning was a boost to my confidence. My roommate, Bruce, was concerned and friendly, and he learned all the signals of an insulin reaction so he could be of help if I ever passed out. I have always been fortunate in that my body can recognize the subtle onset before the violent first wave of an insulin reaction hits me, and I usually dream about it before it actually happens. The dreams are disturbing and I always wake up.

One can never forget diabetes, but when the patient is feeling well he tends to ignore the disease as much as possible. After a few months in Boston, lost in the excitement of a new life and the stimulation of the university, I exercised the minimal requirements of caution, which meant taking my needle in the morning and not much else. This was good for my mind, but murder on my body. I have always thought that the most difficult problem for a diabetic is to achieve a proper balance between mind and body. The two inevitably seem to clash.

Everything was going well. I had been a diabetic for eight years and was functioning much the way I wanted. So I pushed —tempted the disease. I began what I consider the second skirmish in the journey of a diabetic: a battle to see how much the body will tolerate.

I began to stay up late, sure that there were not enough hours in the day, that if I went to sleep I would miss something important. I began to take my insulin irregularly—which causes problems because different types of insulin are effective for different time periods. The action is calibrated so that the mixtures overlap, and fooling with time produces periods of either too much or too little effectiveness. I skipped or delayed meals, which should be timed to coincide with peak insulin hours.

The results were slow, but cumulative in effect, until I reached a point where everything seemed to be falling apart. Diabetes is a degenerative disease, and the process is slow, steady, constant.

It started with a simple infection, an assault on the system by bacteria. The problem for the diabetic is that infection causes the blood sugar to rise, and high sugar makes it harder to fight an invader. This vicious cycle is common in many of the complications of diabetes. I can't even remember what type of infection it was, but suddenly I felt very weak and dizzy, my mouth was dry, and I was urinating a lot. I tried to sleep it off, but only succeeded in making matters worse by missing meals and rising late to take my injections. Finally I realized I would have to see a doctor.

Before I had left New York, Dr. Reese had advised me to go to the Joslin Clinic in Boston, a world-famous institution totally devoted to the treatment of diabetes. I called up and a nurse told me that I would have to wait three months for an appointment. I told her I was feeling very ill, but she replied that they really were booked solid and I would have to wait the three months unless there was a cancellation. I told her I would either be dead or well in three months, and that I would have to look for another doctor.

I still didn't know very much about diabetes at this stage in my life. My faith in doctors was total. I did not ask questions; I was too ignorant and stupid to become involved with my own physical care. Without fully knowing the implications of my disease, I figured that one doctor was as good as the next.

I should have waited the three months.

I walked past a baseball diamond and into a jungle of hospitals and professional buildings. I saw the blue walls of a professional building across the street. Blue has been my favorite color since the age of ten, because the mixture of urine and water will turn deep blue if sugar is not spilling into the bladder from the kidneys. (The renal threshold in relation to blood-sugar levels is 180; if the blood sugar rises above this point, glucose will spill from the kidneys into the bladder. The urine test is a means of keeping track of high sugar levels.)

So I walked into that building only because I liked the color blue, and I gazed at the directory, reading the doctors' names. The one I chose was singled out because his name matched that of one of my favorite pastimes. I will refer to him as Dr. Reading.

It was not the best way to choose a doctor.

In the office the nurse made me fill out forms and said I could see the doctor that same day, but I would have to wait until the other patients in the room had been taken care of. I leafed through several worn issues of *The New Yorker,* a magazine I have always associated with doctors' offices and illness—nothing personal. I glanced at the walls and was impressed by all the framed diplomas. Dr. Reading was a Harvard man. Most of us make a connection between that institution and superior intelligence. The two do not necessarily go together. The city of Boston is filled with Harvard doctors, but in my experience the Ivy League set does not always produce the best physicians. This is no reflection on the institution. I am just trying to make the point that it is important for any person to realize he is dealing with people, not concepts. Intelligence, honesty, and concern depend totally on the person involved, not on affiliations. I could have avoided a lot of pain if I had known this simple fact.

Dr. Reading had a soft, kind voice. The first thing I told him was that I was a diabetic. He said he had treated several diabetics, and that my case would be no problem. It never crossed my mind to ask him if any of those patients was still alive, or if it was going to be no problem for him—or for me.

He said the first thing "we" would do was take a blood test. The office was equipped with a lab, a fact I found impressive because I had never had a blood test on the premises before. I told him that Dr. Reese had always insisted that my blood be drawn early in the morning while fasting, because after meals the level fluctuates and results can vary greatly. He said it "did not make much of a difference," and that the nurse would draw my blood and test it in a few minutes.

It never crossed my mind that this man was not qualified to treat a diabetic, that in reality I had much more experience in dealing with the disease than he did. After all, he had all those diplomas plastered on the wall.

The nurse drew my blood after a few of the usual misses. Back in the examining room, the doctor checked my blood pressure, probed orifices, tested reflexes. He couldn't get my knees to react to his hammer. Then he wrote a prescription for an antibiotic to battle my infection. The nurse came in and handed the doctor a small white piece of paper. I could not see what was written on it.

He looked at the paper for what seemed like a long time, frowning. He told me my blood sugar was fine. I asked him how high it was. He replied again that it was fine. This is an attitude I have encountered many times over the years— one that assumes that we laymen are too ignorant to under- stand the technical jargon of the medical profession. It is a form of intimidation. (I once saw a doctor correct an inter- viewer on television when the man used the term "juvenile diabetic." The doctor said: "Let's get our terms straight, the proper word is juvenile-onset." Well, get this, Doc: I am a person, not an onset.)

Then I was handed the bill: twenty dollars for the office visit *and* twenty for the blood test. I should have known at that moment the real reason why Dr. Reading had set up his own lab. Doctors are just like the rest of us: some are out-and-out greedy. As individuals, some of them are the poorest excuses for human beings I have ever encountered; others are the most noble of men. With Dr. Reading I was guilty of ignorance, but he was guilty of the most callous unconcern.

At the time I hardly realized any of this; I assumed that a doctor was competent just because he was a doctor. So I paid frequent visits to Dr. Reading—an average of once a month. The bad habits of my youth were beginning to catch up with me because of the cumulative nature of the disease. My feet would cramp with such intense pain that many times I could not walk a block without stopping to rest. After some duration, diabetes causes the blood vessels to constrict, impairing circulation, especially to the extremities. There is no known relief for this condition. I would wake in the morning with burning pains in my lower back. Virtually all diabetics suffer from kidney damage of varying severity. Again, there is no known cure.

And Dr. Reading bled me every month, literally and figuratively. He always told me I was fine, and in my stupidity I did not connect the constant pain with the disease, chose not to question the doctor's pronouncements. (I probably didn't want to know what was wrong, to face the reality of the situation.) He never attached a number to my blood-sugar level, as Dr. Reese had always done. Whenever I think of Dr. Reading I am haunted by his one-word vocabulary: *Fine, fine, fine.* And I think of how I was told two days later by another doctor that my blood sugar was so high that I was very close to coma. I become enraged, screaming in my mind: What the hell were you doing with all that blood, you bastard? Spilling it down the drain? Cashing checks and playing with my life? *My life.*

I was under his care for over two years, and never once questioned his approach. The irony is that the Joslin Clinic was practically around the corner, and I had never bothered to return because I thought I was in good hands. Dr. Reading told me that the pain in my back and feet was common for a diabetic. This is true, but his ignorance of the disease set the stage for more serious complications in the future.

My reactions at this stage were typical. I concluded that if there was nothing I could do about the onset of complications, I would at least live my life fully.

As usual, I overreacted.

I stayed up day and night, ignored my diabetes and was filled with the wonders of experimentation. That summer I decided to stay in Boston and see if I could make a living. I was hired as a night cook in a pancake house. I was exhilarated each week when I was handed a paycheck. I thought in some way that I was proving I was a man by fighting the pain in my legs and back. I was drenched from the heat of four large grills, turned thousands of pancakes until I was sick of the sight of them. I got home at four in the morning and tried to wash the smell of bacon from my skin. I was so wound up that I could not sleep for at least three hours. My insulin maintenance and eating habits changed drastically. I was having at least three insulin reactions a night while I was working, and I tried to compensate by drinking a river of Coke every night.

The pain in my legs and back was getting worse, and I was extremely tired all the time. Two deep, purple rings circled my eyes. At times my vision would go out of focus. I went to Dr. Reading and told him I was feeling weak all the time.

The nurse took my blood.

He told me I was fine.

I asked him why I was so tired, why my feet and back hurt all the time.

He asked if I was working.

I told him about my job in the pancake house, of working nights and all the insulin reactions I was getting. I asked him if it might be affecting my diabetes.

He said I was probably just tired and that I should try to get more sleep.

I left and the nurse handed me the bill. I knew I should quit the job, and I had hoped the doctor would tell me that, just as I had always depended on my family and Dr. Reese to give sound advice. In that regard I was partly to blame.

Later on I realized that Dr. Reading didn't really know how to treat a diabetic—in fact, had very little knowledge in the area. He should have known what a shock it was to my system to engage in such heavy work and to keep such late hours, and that my insulin balance was thrown off because of the irregularity of my injections. But he really had no idea of all this.

And he should have uttered those simple words which some doctors find so painful: "I don't know what's wrong; I have very little knowledge of diabetes." Whether the dishonesty of someone like Dr. Reading is motivated by pride or greed makes little difference. I was the one who was getting sicker.

My parents knew I was sick, and they pressured me to come home so I could see Dr. Reese. By this time I could hardly rise in the morning, so I forgot my stubborn dreams and agreed to come home.

The first thing Dr. Reese did was send me to a lab for a blood test. The proper way: after I had taken my insulin and before I had eaten. He was startled when the results came in. My blood-sugar level was over 400. (The normal level is 80 to 120.) He told me I was very close to coma.

My condition was so serious that it was necessary for me to take two needles a day. Thank you, Dr. Reading. I rested and watched myself for a month, and my condition slowly came under control.

Oddly enough, Dr. Reading had taken my blood just two

days before I came home and told me I was fine. Fine is about
150 for a diabetic. I don't think the flight home was responsible
for a rise of over 250 in my blood sugar.

When I returned to Boston, I made a long-overdue phone call
to the Joslin Clinic. This time I waited for the appointment,
despite my habitual impatience.

I have a long-standing grudge with time. Diabetes is a disease
filled with uncertainty, an awareness of crippling complications
that can abort any concept of the future. The possibility that
time may be cut short clouds the mind, squeezes the process of
living. I have tried to stretch time, to live the present moment
to the utmost in an attempt to blunt the terror of what might
lie ahead. I am frightened of the future because it holds the
possibility of sickness and death at any time. This is true for any
person, but the diabetic lives more immediately with these concerns.

I think these fears must have played a large part in my
staying under the care of Dr. Reading for so long. I must have
known deep down that he was not caring for me properly. After
all, I was feeling sick, even if he told me I was well. I should
at least have sought another opinion; I did not. I think that,
subconsciously, I wanted to be told I was well, to hide the
illness so that I did not have to face it.

At the Joslin Clinic, when I finally got there, I felt as though
I were sitting in the lobby of an old-age home. Of all the
diabetics in this country, only 5 percent have the more severe
juvenile type. The curious old-timers always stare at me when
I sit in a waiting room. It's depressing, because they seem to
present a frightening vision of the future. Many older diabetics
suffer greatly, and it is sad to see them complain like terrified
children. The sound of moans is augmented by the drone of
wheelchairs. Many of these people are blind, and they cry when

they are left alone. A good number in the Joslin Clinic were missing arms and legs. Relatives and nurses too often seem weary of them, bored with their suffering. How horrible it must feel to be a burden to loved ones.

I see an image of myself in people like these; I rub my leg and wonder if it will be missing one day. How will I handle these very real losses? Will I be able to live with the pain, and more important, the psychological trauma of physical loss? Will I cry out in a trembling voice until the ones I love, those who have given me the most comfort and care, are sick to death of my complaining? There comes a stage when a diabetic begins to feel concern for the people who will inevitably become tangled in his life. They too sit in doctors' offices and wait.

The doctors at Joslin took me in and examined me. They were honest, listing a host of possible complications. They attached names to the pains in my feet and back (which I will discuss later on), but to my amazement said that they really were not sure what caused them. I was astounded, not by their ignorance, but rather by their simple honest admission of it. I have come to have a great deal of respect for this approach. A person must accept things he cannot control, so that he may concentrate on matters within his grasp.

They talked of kidney damage, heart attack, stroke, blindness, gangrene, arteriosclerosis, acidosis poisoning, infection.

It was not a scare tactic. It was the truth. They told me that good control might help me avoid these complications.

Might.

It is a very hard word to live with. Doctors have argued that good control is the key in handling diabetes. Others say that control really doesn't make a difference. Some researchers have even gone so far as to say that insulin is the cause of diabetic complications. No one really knows the answers.

I do know that I feel better when my sugar is under control. That, for me, is reason enough for control. The struggle to survive is difficult; a good day is a blessing.

I have to live with unanswered questions. While doctors argue at medical conclaves, my own view is very limited. Do I take insulin, and perhaps go blind? Or do I stop the injections, and die? Some choice. Research is valuable when results are obtained. Suspicions complicate my life.

After my visit to the Joslin Clinic I opted for good control and decided I must accept the unanswered questions. To stop fighting. I do not mean total resignation. In fact, it is ironic that the patient takes a more active role in his personal care when he comes to accept his limitations. It is a matter of channeling energy in the right direction. When I gave up on matters outside of my control, I spent a great deal of time trying to maintain a good blood-sugar level. I watched my diet for the first time in my life. I exercised. Good God, I even began to feel healthy.

So I returned to university life with the new attitude that my health was my main concern. I quickly learned that it was not many other people's concern.

My first real clash was with a man I'll call Professor Mortimer, a very minor poet who was teaching a course on the collected works of a major poet. (I think he always resented the fact that it wasn't the other way around.) Mortimer assigned a report based on the reading of about ten books.

I could not even focus on the page, much less read the books.

The doctor at the Joslin Clinic told me that my vision was changing due to the onset of retinopathy. This disease (which I'll discuss in more detail in a later chapter) is a leading cause of blindness. The blood vessels of the retina dilate and burst, blocking the retina; if enough vessels burst, the patient goes blind.

The doctor said that a few of my blood vessels had burst, and that this was the cause of my problem. He said that my condition was not severe at this time, and that my inability to focus would most likely clear up. He simply advised me not to read until my eyes felt better.

I told all this to Mortimer and assured him that somehow I would manage to complete the work. He answered that if I couldn't do the work on time I should get out of his course. He did have a point. I imagine that the university was his life, and he chose not to bend the rules and regulations of that community. I could not read the books; I could not do the work. Simple, rational facts. My personal concerns were but a speck in his universe.

But it was too late in the semester to enroll in a different course, so I would lose the four credits and have to make them up some other time—a threat to graduation. I had never been asked to leave a course.

Mortimer said he would not tolerate excuses, and that he expected his work to be done.

It struck home that it was my *eyes* that were in question. *My eyes.* And I thought of all the years I had neglected my health, of the price I was beginning to pay. And I saw that my vision was of no concern to Mortimer, that he was caught up in playing academic games and would not back down on his fixed demands, no matter what the reason.

I felt great anger: rage that this man could care so little for the well-being of another human. A simple thought crossed my mind: Screw you, Mortimer. If you don't care, at least I do.

I began to scream at him, but my anger was tinged with an inner feeling of warmth, the security of knowing that at least *I* cared. "You bastard," I said, "take your course and shove it."

I told him I would not drop the course, and that if he tried to kick me out, I would fight all the way up to the president of the university. I said my health was more important than his rules, and that I would finish the report when my eyes were better.

He was silent for a long time. "You're not a competent student," he said.

I began to laugh. "You're not a competent human being," I said. "And I really don't care what you think of me."

He sat there, stunned. And then I uttered the words I found so satisfying at the time, words that lifted a great weight that had accumulated over the years. I said it out loud this time: "Screw you, Mortimer."

I said it again, louder. Mortimer was quiet.

No one could care for my body as I could myself. I would have to stand up and fight for it.

Mortimer never did try to remove me from the seminar. For once in my life, *I* was in control.

7

The Absurdity of Death

MY SUGAR WAS RISING, a not uncommon situation for me, but this time I was at a loss to understand it. There was the parched mouth, weakness, aches, boils, excessive, burning urination—a frightening setback because it defied logic. I was finally taking care of myself, yet was feeling like that confused, sickly child of ten.

My father, an astute businessman with a keen eye for the subtle changes of the stock market, told me once that when my sugar went over 400 I should sell.

I wish I had such an option. The disease has been recorded and described for close to 3500 years; the cause is *still* a mystery. The medical world knows only the effects of complications, and a definite relation to the disease has been established by observation, but the process of degeneration and means of prevention are barely understood. Insulin plays a role in balancing blood-sugar levels, but the complex nature of its action is unknown. It is not a cure. I myself consider insulin no more than a reprieve.

On December 10, 1975, the National Commission on Diabetes presented a report to Congress that was crucial in convincing the government and public of the need for research. The most striking feature of the paper was the lengthy listing of severe complications that most diabetics suffer from, coupled with the astounding admission of the lack of knowledge in all of these areas. The report was both frightening and heartening (more about it later).

Several years before this report was released, I experienced an intimate relationship with one of the complications it listed.

How can I communicate the pure terror of waking in the middle of the night and having no sensation in my feet, of looking down and praying that they might still be there? Or the constant, burning pain in my lower back? And the ache, the gnawing weakness that seemed to cry, "Give up, give up" a hundred times a day. Over and over I repeated the same question: What is the cause?

With the steady rise in sugar, I realized that proper diet and insulin maintenance were not always enough.

At the Joslin Clinic, the doctor was at a loss to explain my condition. My sugar was indeed high, near the point at which my father had advised selling, but all the doctor could speculate was that I was suffering from some infection. But you cannot treat an unknown factor. We agreed that all we could do was watch and wait—yes, agreed. I think the most important factor about the Joslin Clinic is that the patient is encouraged to become involved in his treatment. The doctors there realize that the diabetic has a great deal of expertise in dealing with his own body. The approach hinges on the concept of a responsible patient, which is in fact the key to living with diabetes.

I watched. Waited. Even prayed.

Nothing happened. I prayed some more. I have had my problems with the Creator, but have always turned to Him in times of stress. That summer I was going downhill fast: for a month I was very close to setting an all-time personal record for high blood sugar.

Then, by accident, the invader was exposed, the mystery solved on a visit to the dentist for a routine six-month examination.

The dentist probed my mouth, then paused, and his expression turned serious. He told me to open my mouth as wide as possible, and he jabbed at the back with a long, thin steel instrument. I felt a sharp pain but could not place it.

It turned out that my four wisdom teeth were infected. He also said that my bone structure was very weak and the molars were brittle. He probed again and a piece of my tooth disintegrated.

I called my doctor at the Joslin Clinic, and he told me that infected teeth often throw control off balance. He said I should have them pulled as soon as possible, but that I should try to get my sugar down before having the extractions. Any such shock to the body causes the sugar to rise, and my level was already too high.

My problem: to get the sugar down because the teeth were getting it up, but the sugar would not go down because the teeth were infected, and the teeth could not be pulled because the sugar was too high, and the sugar was too high because the teeth were infected . . .

The seeming hopelessness of it all resulted in a setback in attitude. I decided that if matters were going to be so absurd, I would ignore them for a time and concentrate on something I considered very important. Looking back now, I realize it was the worst, and the best, thing I could have done.

A distinguished novelist is indirectly responsible for my

nutty behavior, though he has never had any idea of how he influenced me. John Cheever has been for many years my favorite American writer, and as it happened, at the time my teeth were bombarding my system the announcement was made that Cheever was coming to teach a seminar at Boston University. I decided that nothing—my experience with Professor Mortimer notwithstanding—would stop me from becoming a member of that class. The procedure was for each student to write a short story and Cheever would decide, on reading them, whom he wanted in the class.

I decided to forget my teeth for a time and concentrate on writing a story. It took six long weeks, a time filled with weakness, pain, and an intense desire to create good fiction. Several mornings I woke with shattered bits of tooth on my palate. It seems crazy now, but I had a great need to write that story. It was about a man whose world did not unfold according to his vision of it, a man who longed for the past. I have no idea now why I wrote such a story, what intrigued me about this longing for the past.

For two weeks after turning in my story I waited for the Cheever class list to be posted in the English department. I would pace the green along the Charles River to gather courage as each day passed without the posting.

Then I saw my name. It was a moment of great joy, but at the same time I realized that my body was in such need of attention that if I did not act soon I might never sit in that seminar. I was losing weight; the sugar was still rising. The pain in my legs and back was constant. The absurd yet frightening truth was that my life now depended on the extraction of those infected teeth.

It was time again to fly home to Dr. Reese. He immediately put me on a strict diet. But the infected teeth would not let up, and my sugar would not go down. All the old fears returned. I was feeling very sick, and at such times the idea of dying infects the mind. My condition was serious, though I am not actually sure that the situation could have proven fatal. Still, no one should have to see death in the space of four molars.

As always, I turned to Freddy, with whom I had maintained a close relationship since our summer camp days. We took endless walks, sat in bars for hours, and talked constantly. I touched nothing stronger than club soda. I talked of how frustrating the dental situation was, of how all my attempts at lowering my sugar level had failed. Most of all, I talked of the impotent feeling of living with a body that went out of control for the slightest of reasons. I could not understand it; that was the hardest thing to live with.

Freddy could only listen. But it was enough to have someone who understood, even if he was powerless to help.

Dr. Reese finally acknowledged that there was no likelihood my sugar would go down. I would have to risk having the teeth pulled as things were.

I was referred to a dentist. His walls were filled with framed newspaper clippings, yellow with age. In all the photos, a man in an army uniform (a young version of the dentist) stood next to President Roosevelt. The nurse told me that the doctor had pulled out one of F.D.R.'s teeth during the war. I imagine the pictures were supposed to convince the patients that they were in good hands; or perhaps the dentist was simply proud of his association with the President.

The dentist had a long phone conversation with Dr. Reese. They decided that I could not be given general anesthesia during the extractions, in case anything went wrong. I would be given a shot of Novocain during the process, but could not take any painkillers afterward.

I had never had anything removed from my body before, and I was nervous and apprehensive about the whole thing.

The dentist remarked that my teeth were quite brittle and that the connective tissue and bone were wearing away. He advised that I have two of the teeth removed, then come back another day to finish off the job. I thought, mostly because of my fear, that it would be better to take out all four at once. It had been hard enough to get this far. I did not want to come back again. So I sat in the chair, gripping the armrests until my knuckles turned white.

After injecting Novocain and waiting for it to take effect, he took a scooplike instrument that he put between my gums and the base of the tooth. It acted like a lever, and when he pushed down I felt a great pressure rising in my mouth, then tasted blood.

A sharp pain traveled in circles around my mouth. My chin was numb, but I could feel blood oozing down my neck. The pressure would not stop.

Next, he gripped the tooth with a long pliers. He pulled. Nothing budged. The Novocain was not working very well.

He raised his leg, resting it on the chair between the V of my crotch. Careful, I thought. He put his open palm on the center of my forehead and pressed down. Then he pushed back, tensed his leg, and pulled. And pulled. And pulled.

The tooth shattered. My mouth was filled with bits of bone. The explosion sent them down my throat. I began to choke on a combination of bone and blood.

The dentist cursed, then muttered that I was giving him a lot of trouble. I wondered if Roosevelt had caused him such problems.

He moved away for a moment, came back with a thinner

pliers. He told me that the tooth was too brittle, that it had shattered and snapped from the root.

He put his palm on my forehead again. It was wet with perspiration. He began to dig with the long pliers. I averted my eyes from the white bits he was removing from my mouth.

As he went deeper, the pain became more intense. I felt the blood drying on my neck. He pulled again, and I felt the same rising pressure. The root came out. He began to dig to make sure all the shattered bits of bone were removed. He started digging at my tongue and at the back of my throat, sifting through the wreckage of my former tooth.

The nurse came with a suction instrument and vacuumed the bone and blood from my mouth.

Three more to go, said the dentist.

The same thing happened with the other teeth. All of them shattered. First the explosion, then the river of blood flowing from my mouth.

The dentist remarked that he had never had such a hard time pulling teeth. He had pulled the former President's tooth, he said, in a few minutes. That answered my question.

My mouth cost him about three hours. Why couldn't I have normal molars? The futile wish of a diabetic.

At home, the Novocain wore off. I couldn't sleep for the constant pain, but there was nothing I could take to ease the suffering. Large blood clots broke from the tooth spaces; I packed my mouth with wads of cotton to try to stem the bleeding.

I gagged on clots for about a week, swallowed them, and woke with the foul odor of dried blood in my mouth. Then I vomited the blood from my stomach.

My whole mouth was so sore I couldn't eat solid food. My sugar began to go down, but still I could not eat. I was getting insulin reactions again, and I greeted them with a mixture of gratitude and fright—at least my sugar was going down. My mother mashed all kinds of things in the blender so that I began to get food down. I took a little less insulin. I finally gained some measure of control.

I would later learn from the National Commission on Diabetes report that peridontal disease is a common complication of diabetes. The report stated:

> The incidence of serious peridontal disease among individuals with diabetes is estimated to be as much as three times higher than among normal individuals. Generally the disease is more serious and progresses more rapidly in diabetic patients. . . . Periodontal disease causes serious difficulties in mastication and other discomforts and problems such as *infection.* [Italics added.]

The cause of the problem, again, is a mystery. The disease brings on the deterioration of dental bones, and the teeth become dislodged. It is believed that diabetics have a predisposition to a loss of bone throughout the body.

I went back to Boston with a new sense of the fragility and absurdity of my body. I knew now how serious my condition could become for the smallest of reasons. If teeth could get you, anything was possible. It was a paranoiac view of life, but the dangers were real. The problem was to come to terms with these new fears.

As a diabetic, I could not fight against the workings of my body. I could exercise caution, and seek medical attention when necessary, but I could not stop the degenerative processes of my disease. So there comes another emotion, though it is not exclusively confined to diabetes: powerlessness. The only way to fight is to sit back, but never give in. Emotional turmoil runs high until the diabetic learns that he must accept many aspects of his condition. A person can go mad if he tries to find a reason for all of his suffering.

I will never sit back and give in to my disease, but I will not engage in useless skirmishes. Life is complex, with various goals and aspirations. I will not spend my life cursing my teeth, because I would use up precious energy. I can now look back and laugh about the episode—because diabetes is only a part of my life, not all of it.

I will always take care of my body, watch it like a faithful lover. But I will not live as if I have one foot in the grave, because that is so barren a concept that it rules out the possibility of joy and fulfillment. Ironically, this attitude develops only after one realizes and accepts the extent of his powerlessness. Only then can he move on to other matters.

It was fortunate that I reached this understanding in the middle of John Cheever's fiction seminar. He asked us to keep a journal and bring it in for the next session. My first impression was that he was a man who understood many things, so I decided to deal with my diabetes in the journal. I wrote about all the matters weighing on my mind. It was a revelation to see my honest reactions on paper; it gave me a certain sense of distance.

But while I was writing, I did not consider that I would be reciting all this in front of strangers. I was terrified as we sat around the large white table in the classroom. I was one of the last to read my journal. Many of the other students had written of getting drunk or of trying to crash a baseball game in Fenway Park. Few of them dealt with matters of a personal nature. It had been a simple exercise to write down all my thoughts and related fears—it was another matter to read them to a class full of strangers. There was no backing down. My voice cracked as

I started to read, and several of the students laughed. My
stomach was queasy through the entire reading; my voice trem-
bled. My soaked hands stuck to the pages.

Some excerpts:

> At the proper moment I plunge the needle forward—hesitate at
> the last second—then pushing slowly the skin caves in and I feel
> a tinge of pain as it slides slowly into my flesh. It would be better
> not to hesitate, but something always makes me slow down.
> Perhaps it's the expectation, the knowledge of what this all
> means.

I revealed one of my secrets concerning the fear of death,
something I had only discussed with Freddy:

> The possibility of death frightens me. I don't think it's the fact
> of dying, but rather the uncertainty, the ambiguity as to the time
> remaining.

On the fear of blindness:

> A thought has just occurred: if I go blind, will I be able to detect
> the presence of great works of art by my sense of smell, and if
> so, will the odor of a painting by Michelangelo be overpowered
> by the unshaven armpits of Italian women? In this respect, is Art
> more powerful than life?

And I wrote of the sense of frustration I had suffered because
of my disease:

> I have the need for a place in the realm of Time and Space, for
> a moment of pure certainty. Even wasps and field mice have that
> second, that instant of balanced quietude.

The room was quiet for what seemed like a long time. I
looked down at the table and tried to stop trembling. Then I
raised my head and looked into Cheever's face. He smiled.

He uttered a single word: "Marvelous."

I felt a lifting, a cleansing of wounds. I had bared my feelings and had not been scorned.

I learned to rejoice that day, to value the power of understanding and concern, and if I had suffered because of teeth and needle, pain and weakness, I also learned the awesome pleasure contained in the simple fact of being alive.

8

Vision

I AM AFRAID of going blind. When I wake in the morning I look out the window at things I may someday see no more—autumn leaves, an expanse of lawn, a flock of birds. Indoors, I gaze at pictures, at books, even at ashtrays, to make sure I will always remember what they look like.

The fear presses on my mind every day of my life. Profoundly depressed, I sit at a typewriter and wonder if I would be able to manage simple tasks without the use of my eyes.

My fears are not groundless. Diabetics are twenty-five times more likely to go blind than nondiabetics, according to the National Commission on Diabetes. (Other researchers' figures vary slightly, depending on the source; none of them is comforting.) Diabetes is known to be the leading cause of blindness in adults. It has been estimated that 80 percent of *all* diabetics suffer eye damage; among juvenile diabetics, the complications are more severe.

If a diabetic goes blind, he will not know the specific reason, except that it is an expected complication of the disease. But there are no real answers. We can only sit back and hope to be spared; we cannot fight a mystery. Perhaps someday it will be solved. Meanwhile, there are various forms of treatment, most of them controversial, but there is no way to prevent the problems because there is no understanding of the cause.

At the root of the problem is a disease called diabetic retinopathy. It is closely related to the changes in the vascular system that play a crucial role in diabetic complications. *Something* causes changes in the small blood vessels of the eye, and as a result these vessels dilate and burst, blocking vision. The retina often becomes detached; clogged vessels often grow out in other directions, clouding sight. The result is impaired vision —or blindness.

Some diabetics are spared the complications of retinopathy. No one knows why; as yet it has not been determined that there is any relationship between good control and the onset of retinopathy. The changes occur slowly, steadily—a constant reminder of the fragility of a diabetic's life.

A diabetic will inevitably have bouts with uncontrollable forces in his body, and he needs to be able to face them. It can be devastating to have to face the truth suddenly. Recognition can be a great source of comfort, even if nothing can be changed. It is best to be prepared when the collector comes to call, not because the price will be lower, but to give yourself time to come to terms with the magnitude of his bills.

From the day that the onset of retinopathy caused me problems with Professor Mortimer, the disease became a constant burden on my mind.

I visit the eye doctor twice a year. It is always a traumatic experience. Dr. Oculus is a busy man who is probably very dedicated to his work. But he is also inconsiderate. I think he must view his patients as specimens. I have been degraded and beaten enough by my body. I resent that kind of treatment from a doctor. If he can't offer a cure, why can he not at least offer a little comfort?

The nurse leads me down a long corridor and places drops in my eyes to dilate the pupils. I always walk outside for some air, and squint from the bright glare of the sun. I keep my eyes trained on the ground.

On these walks I often encounter the relative of a diabetic. On one occasion, though I could not focus on the man's face, I could hear the unmistakable trembling in his voice. He told me that his son, at twenty-eight, was going blind. Dr. Oculus had given him that news as if he were ticking off a stock quotation; the doctor did not have to deal with the problem personally. The man talked of his own frustration and guilt, of his powerlessness to help his own flesh and blood. He had had to sit back, he told me, and watch his son's world disappear. He blamed himself because of the history of diabetes on his side of the family. He clenched his fists and cried.

I tried to tell him that there could have been no way of knowing that his child would lose his sight one day. I said all the expected things: that one might die at any time, be hit by a car or pushed onto the subway tracks. What I said did not help. I myself had never been comforted by any of the rationalizations that had been offered me.

I watched the man leave, leading his son by the arm, and I grieved for the pain and loss that parents must endure when children suffer so senselessly.

Another day, I saw a man turned away from the office because he could not afford laser treatments. He had the powerfully built, squat frame of a laborer. He was wearing a worn, checkered coat and his face was covered with stubble. He told the nurse he did not have insurance; he could not afford *five hundred dollars* per treatment. He asked if he could pay in installments. The nurse said that all bills were to be settled before treatment. (Much later, I learned that Dr. Oculus would treat patients for free at a hospital clinic, but the nurse never mentioned this fact.) The man started to beg, said he would go blind without the treatments. The nurse walked away.

I know the argument: if you give it away for free, people will start taking advantage of you. But I could not imagine Dr. Oculus starving to death. He does a six-figure business annually in Medicaid alone. I could understand the man's predicament: were it not for my parents, I could not have afforded this doctor either. Diabetes is expensive. Vision is priceless.

Since the blood vessels in my eyes were beginning to burst, I was a frequent visitor to Dr. Oculus. He said there was nothing to be done at this stage, that the condition was not yet bad enough to warrant laser treatment.

I asked him if I might go blind.

He said yes.

Dr. Oculus does not have a refined bedside manner. As many times as I've seen him, I have often put my hand forward in greeting, but he has always ignored it. Perhaps he has bad eyes. He certainly ignores questions, and frowns on jokes during an examination.

At some point during my bout with retinopathy he decided that I should undergo a test called a fluorescein angiograph. This involves the injection of a red dye that travels to the blood vessels of the eye. Pictures are taken in rapid succession to determine the extent of the damage from leaking vessels.

The nurse said to come in the next day and to bring $125 for the test.

After she had put drops in my eyes, the nurse asked me to sign a form. I told her I could not read the paper.

She said it was the usual form.

I asked her what that meant.

She said I was being difficult.

I told her I only wanted to know what the paper said.

She said it was a standard form, absolving the doctor of responsibility for any side effects from the test.

There had been no mention of side effects the day before, only of money.

I got angry, and told the nurse I wanted to know exactly what was going on. If they didn't care about my eyes or my health, they could at least have the decency to tell me what was involved in the test. I said that if I was going to take risks, I wanted to be informed of what they were.

She told me I did not have much choice in the matter: if I refused to have the test, the doctor could not tell what was wrong with my eyes.

They always do have the upper hand.

I asked again about the side effects.

The dye, she said, would make my skin turn yellow for a few days, and my urine would be discolored.

Since I had never been vain about my complexion, I told her I would take the test but did not want to sign the paper.

No signature, no test.

I signed the release. I should have been even more suspicious than I was.

She took me to a room where I was sat down before a huge mass of steel. A camera was strapped to the back of the machine. On the table rested a syringe with a long coil. A needle was attached to the end of the coil. A red substance filled the syringe.

Another nurse came in and explained that my head would be placed against the brace in the center of the machine. The dye would be injected into a vein in my arm and rush to my eyes, within five seconds. In the photographs, the dye would reveal the extent of bleeding and retinal damage.

She began a search for my hard-to-find veins. Each time she missed, she became more frustrated, then angry. She had never seen such bad veins, she told me.

I apologized for being uncooperative. My veins, I told her, would never listen to me.

Without answering, she left the room for several minutes. She returned with Dr. Oculus.

"What's the problem here?" he asked.

I told him about the nurse's inability to find a vein.

"Let me have a look," he said.

I offered my arm and he made a long inspection. Then he raised the needle and aimed it.

Laughing, I asked him if my elbow would turn red from the dye if he missed the vein.

He did not find my comment amusing. He never missed, he told me. I said I had just been trying to ease the tension.

Dr. Oculus said that no one in his office was tense.

No one who works for you, I thought. Just the patients.

He hit a vein, all right, but did not inject the dye. He left the room telling the nurse that everything was ready.

She began a check of the machine. I asked her if there was film in the camera. She put my head against the brace and her hand on the plunger of the syringe.

She flicked a switch and a blue beam of light began to pulse at regular intervals. My dilated eyes started aching from the intensity of the light.

"Don't move," she told me.

She pushed the plunger. My ears were bombarded by lightning clicks of the camera.

I felt the invader rush through my system—and suddenly intense pressure in my head. My tongue and eyes seemed to be swelling, my nose was filled with blood. My entire head throbbed in anticipated explosion.

I thought I was going to pass out. "I feel sick," I said, the sound of the camera pounding in my ears.

The nurse told me not to move. She said the dye was responsible for whatever I was feeling. If I moved I would ruin the whole test, she said.

I told her I thought I was going to pass out.

"Hold on just a few more seconds."

The sensation of pressure seemed to be concentrating in my nose. I was going to sneeze, I told the nurse.

Was she screaming, or was I only imagining it? She said I would ruin the test if I sneezed, that all this equipment was terribly expensive and *she* would be responsible if I mucked up the test. I wondered what was more valuable than my eyes.

It was over finally. I had to be helped out of the room, to sit down for at least an hour. I asked the nurse why I had not been warned about my possible reaction. She said they did not want to worry patients. I told her that if I had been warned, I would have brought someone along to help me home.

They had never thought of that. Dr. Oculus and his band of nurses did not have to worry about my getting home. That was my problem. So was the reaction. So was blindness.

I went home and pissed orange for three days. Everyone said I had a nice tan.

My eyes were leaking, but not severely. A year later, all signs of retinopathy had disappeared. Dr. Oculus offered me no real or fancied explanation. I knew the disease could return at any time, but I rejoiced.

I did not ask questions.

9

Painful Steps

SO FAR I HAVE BEEN DEALING, for the most part, with the upper regions of my body—eyes, teeth, and mind. Let me take you now on a severe plunge downward, past some of the complicated network of the circulatory system, through the pounding of my heart. We will weave through the tangle of peripheral nerves running down the spinal cord, past the kidneys and other vital organs. Forget for a moment that the landscape has been ravaged.

Farther on, the complex highway we are traveling narrows and branches into endless country roads. The paths are clogged, and progress becomes slow. Near the end of the trek, at the base of one foot, traffic is altogether snarled. There is an obstruction in the middle of the road. It is tough, hard as a rock. It dams and slows the flow of blood, and causes a great deal of pain alternating with the loss of sensation.

A wart. Diabetes does not cause warts. But a wart on the ball of a diabetic's foot can create untold dangers.

The wart had been growing steadily for two years, and by now it felt as if a nail was embedded in my foot. My feet had always been a problem because of poor circulation and nerve damage; they often caused me pain, and at times had become numb. Concerned with the wart, I finally showed it to my doctor at the Joslin Clinic. He said it was a common seeded wart, and that at this stage I should leave it alone.

Feet are of crucial concern to a diabetic. The loss of circulation means that the body's defense mechanisms cannot reach the area; and that waste products cannot be washed away through the blood. Since the body cannot fight infection in the area, healing is slow, and wounds can remain open for long periods.

Moreover, impaired circulation creates the danger of gangrene. Diabetes is a major factor in the spread of gangrene. That means amputation. I have sat in too many waiting rooms with people who have missing limbs.

The clinic doctor thought it best to leave the wart alone because he knew the danger of an open wound that might not heal. But the wart spread, until every step became a painful limp. So I went back to see Dr. Reese. He was afraid that it might become infected; but either way, there was danger involved. I decided to have the wart removed, so Dr. Reese gave me the name of a podiatrist, whom I'll call Dr. Plantar, after the type of growth on my foot.

The doctor's office was jammed with patients, and people were exiting from the examining room at five-minute intervals. Obviously, he was a practitioner of the quick-turnover theory of medicine. I waited for about an hour until the nurse led me into the doctor's office. Dr. Plantar was sitting behind a huge wooden desk; papers were scattered along the surface, and there were actually dust balls clinging to one large stack of papers.

I remember what I said, because it is the first thing I always say: "I'm a diabetic."

He made no answer to that—which should have been my cue to leave his office immediately. After I told him I had a wart on the bottom of my foot, he said to take off my shoe and sock and put my foot on the desk. No examining room?

He looked at my foot for not more than five seconds, and did not even touch the growth. He just nodded his head.

I told him I was concerned because of the poor circulation in my feet.

"This is nothing," said Plantar. "It's just a common seeded wart."

On a sheet of paper, he drew a pyramid. Pointing with a pencil, he explained that the wart spread out as it grew deeper.

He said we would burn it with acid and then cut it out. I have learned to become suspicious when doctors say "we."

"I want you to buy salicylic acid," he said. "It's a paste. Put it on the wart and cover it with a bandage. Leave it on for a week."

I reminded him that I was a diabetic.

"We do this all the time," he told me, and said that the acid would burn away the wart. After a week the skin would be dead. I was then to take off the bandage and slice off the dead skin with a knife.

He told me to repeat the procedure every week until I had burned and sliced off the entire wart. It would take about six weeks.

I commented that it sounded as if I would be cutting off most of my foot.

"We do this all the time," he said.

On my first visit to the Joslin Clinic, I had been told that the feet were an area of such concern that I should exercise extreme caution even when cutting my toenails—lacerations simply could not be trusted to heal. My poor cat had to give up his claws, against his will, because he once made four long gashes on my foot. The scabs took four months to heal.

I told all this to Dr. Plantar. He said I was overreacting. I had the impression that he wanted me out of his office, that I was taking up too much of his time. Money and time often pose a dual problem for the chronically ill. We spend a great deal of money on medical attention, but it often seems to me that we get very little time for it.

The time part of the equation was over in less than ten minutes; now for the money. I walked over to the front desk. The nurse, a huge woman, had hair that matched the starched white of her uniform. She was one of those seasoned hard and bitter people who seem to be tired of dealing with sickness, not because they feel for the patients, but because they resent having to hear the constant drone of illness. This one, I thought, really looked like a mean old bitch.

I was right.

She ignored me for a long time, a common tactic. My entire consultation with the doctor had taken less time than my waiting now for the nurse. When she did finally turn to me, she got right down to business: "Thirty-five dollars," she said.

I panicked. I had a total of twenty-five dollars in my wallet. My checking account, which was rarely a source of comfort, was dry.

I asked the nurse to bill me.

She took a cardboard sign from under the desk: ALL BILLS WILL BE SETTLED AT TIME OF VISIT.

I told her I had never been able to see through walls. She did not find the remark amusing.

"You have to pay the bill before you leave," she said angrily. "Thirty-five dollars."

I told her that she should have informed me of this over the phone when I made the appointment, that I did not have that amount of money with me.

Her response was very loud: "I always have at least that much with me. How could you go to the doctor without money?"

Every head in the waiting room turned toward me. I was embarrassed and angry. I asked her again to give me a bill.

"If you don't have the money, how do I know you'll send it in?" she asked. And then again, loudly: "*I* always have money on *me.*"

"Then why don't you pay my bill?" I suggested.

"All bills have to be settled," she said. "It's policy."

I told her again that I hadn't known how much the doctor would charge.

"Dr. Plantar is very reasonable," she said.

"For ten minutes? He didn't even examine me," I said.

"That is not the issue," she said.

I told her that I was not going to argue, that either she would give me a bill or I was going to walk out.

Muttering something about never seeing the money, she threw the bill over the desk.

I go into the details of this episode because of the important role that kind of attitude plays in the diabetic's life. While the nurse worried about getting my money, I was worried about the possibility of losing my foot. I realize health care is a business, but I don't think it fair to subject the patient to intimidation and embarrassment.

Perhaps I overreact. But if you were told on April 15 that you or a loved one had cancer, I doubt that you would spend the day worrying about your taxes.

Diabetes is an expensive disease. Its cost for all the sufferers in the United States—without considering the cost of its complications—is estimated at more than $5 billion a year. There are no price controls on insulin. In the fifteen years I have had diabetes, the cost of insulin has risen about *300 percent.* A diabetic cannot boycott insulin.

I do not fault a doctor for wanting to be paid. I simply want my health to be the primary thing on his mind. Dr. Plantar said he was not worried about me. I was. And his ignorance of diabetic problems caused my life to turn into a nightmare.

Yet now I blame myself a great deal for what happened in Plantar's office. Too often, we exercise more care in selecting a car than a doctor. It is I who hold the responsibility for the care of my body, and I think this is the single most important fact to be recognized in the life of a diabetic (or anyone, for that matter). We must come to realize that no one will ever be more concerned than we are.

I went home, and the first thing I did was send in payment of the bill. Then I went to a drugstore and bought the salicylic acid and a special knife to slice off the dead skin. On the street I opened the white bag and removed the box of acid. I read the long list of cautions, and near the bottom I saw the words: *Not for use by diabetics.*

I cursed and limped back toward home. I saw children running in the park and thought of the simple pleasure of moving around without pain. Then I sat on a bench for a long time, watching some young boys playing basketball, enchanted by the graceful motion of limbs, the coiled tension of muscular bodies. I watched them as a fight broke out—the easy anger of youth in competition—and I wanted to interrupt, to tell them how much they should enjoy the fantastic magic of movement.

I walked into my apartment and called Dr. Reese. I told him everything about my visit to Dr. Plantar, including the warning on the box of acid. He said to try one application of the acid and see if it helped. (He knew of no other podiatrists I could consult.)

I was scared by both the wart and the medicine. I have dreamed of seeing a few simple words printed on a medicine label: *Specially formulated for diabetics. Abandon caution for once in your life and relax.*

I opened the box.

The acid was a dried white paste attached to a gauze backing. I cut out a circle about the size of a penny—the same size as the exposed portion of the wart. I imagined burning a hole in my foot, and suddenly another image came back to haunt me: the child burning in the house of God. Visions of the past; the return of old connections. The absurdity of death and feet; the absurdity of death and teeth.

I followed the instructions and put the acid pad on the sole of my foot, then wrapped a bandage around it.

All I could do now was wait. It was a week of burning pain, burning doubt.

I removed the bandage, and my nose was assaulted by that horrible smell of burned flesh. I twisted my foot and forced myself to look down. I turned away, frightened by the sight.

The skin was green, moldy, dead. There were burns on the healthy tissue surrounding the wart. The odor was sickening.

I thought for sure that I was going to lose my foot. The pain was actually worse than before. I lifted the knife and stared at it for minutes. The whole procedure seemed so insane to me. I thought of calling Dr. Plantar and asking him if he could slice off the skin, but then decided I did not want the man to touch me. I could imagine him cutting off half my foot in less than thirty seconds, then calling in the next patient.

The whole area around the wart was so sensitive that I gasped at just the touch of the cold steel against my skin.

I waited. I did not want to cut.

The first shaving motion produced a spreading pain deep inside my foot. Since tissue around the wart was swollen and red, I thought it must be infected from the acid, but the source of the pain was much deeper.

I began to slice slowly—a meat cutter, shaving off pieces of my own flesh.

My body began to tremble from the pain; sweat ran down my forehead and into my eyes. I could not hold the knife steady any longer, so I waited.

Then, gritting my teeth, I began again, slowly, painfully slicing off the dead skin. I shaved away for at least an hour. I was now below the level of the healthy tissue, had dug a small crater where the surface of the wart had been. I could not see the end of the dead skin. Going deeper and deeper, I was so far in that I had to use the knife like a scoop. The circumference of the wart only increased as I cut.

I finally stopped because I was afraid I would never reach the end. My whole foot pulsed with pain. I took the knife and acid and threw them in the garbage.

The wart eventually grew back to twice its original size, and walking was more painful for me than ever. Regressing to childhood, I kept my mouth shut. I had sought help, and the treatment had only made matters worse.

I did not seek out another doctor, as foolish as it may sound, for over a year. My loss of faith in the medical profession, together with the frustration of having simple matters become complex problems, created a sense of despair and aloneness. I would rather endure the pain in my foot, which I came to view as inevitable, than see another bumbling doctor. I was, of course, guilty of stereotyping all physicians. Pain has a way of wearing down one's resistance, though, and after silently cursing the foot for a year I finally decided to seek other help.

My mother remembered the name of a surgeon who had once removed a wart from my brother's leg. When I finally went to see this man, he impressed me with his kindness and concern. Putting me on an examining table, he prodded the wart with his fingers. I said I was a diabetic and that I was afraid of gangrene. I told him about the rush job in Plantar's office, the caution on the acid, the knife.

He said the man was insane. He even said that a podiatrist should never have touched my foot, that this type of problem should have been handled surgically to start with. He confirmed my suspicion that the wart had spread and become infected *because* of the acid. Plantar, he said, should have his license taken away; his anger was genuine.

He told me his treatment would take a long time because of the damage from the acid. He wanted to proceed carefully because of my reduced capacity to heal. He was going to give me injections of a substance that would separate the wart from the healthy tissue, then he would remove the wart with an electric needle. He made no mention of gangrene.

He pulled out a long, thick needle. He told me the injection would be painful, and asked if I wanted to be held down. I said no.

He had a hard time breaking the skin. He pushed the needle slowly; it took a long time for the thick liquid to be expelled.

It was the most intense pain I have ever felt in my life.

He finally pulled out the needle, remarking that I was the first patient who had never moved or said a word during that type of injection.

I told him that I was used to dealing with pain and had learned to keep my mouth shut. I talked about the countless people I had heard moaning in waiting rooms, and of my realization that a person suffers alone much of the time, that he has to learn to deal with pain in solitude because other people feel uncomfortable discussing it.

He told me he understood.

For two days after the injection, I limped worse than usual. I went for an injection every week for two months. The medication was painful, but the doctor said the wart was separating nicely. From things he asked, I knew he feared complicating factors, even though we never talked about them.

After the two months of injections, he took an electric needle and carefully burned away, deep into the wart. Again, there was the sickening smell of charred flesh. I prayed that this would be the last time I ever encountered that odor.

The doctor took a scalpel and sliced off a small portion of skin on the surface of the wart. He looked at the area and said that the wart had separated. With a tweezerlike instrument he reached in and simply lifted out the wart. It was about an inch long.

Suddenly the doctor seemed concerned. He told me that the wound was filled with pus. He would have to leave the wound open and let the pus drain out. I instantly thought of gangrene. He put a dressing of cotton into the hole and told me to change it every two days.

I walked, or rather limped, with an open hole in my foot for over two weeks. Yellow pus oozed thickly out of the wound.

The doctor put me on antibiotics. I saw the look on his face; he too was afraid of gangrene.

After a few weeks the pus slowed, and the doctor said I was out of danger.

The wart was removed over four years ago. The hole in my foot is still there.

10

Peripheral Vision

I TRY TO CONTROL my temper. When I start to get angry, I go into my study and close the door, sit perfectly still, and try to relax my muscles. I stare at things—usually the high stacks of books on my desk. I think of what's in them, the order and logic of the universe. If I stay angry, I feel a pounding in my head —high blood pressure. I begin to breathe heavily and there is a sour taste in my mouth. I can actually feel my sugar rising. I want to stop it, but it is now too late to control my reaction. My mouth gets dry, and I gulp down huge amounts of water. Fatigue spreads to every corner of my body. I want to sleep, but can't. I shuttle to the bathroom most of the night. *Now I am truly enraged—because I cannot control my rage.* It makes my sugar rise, makes me feel sick. The lack of control is now critical.

I do not often become angry with people. I have learned to respect different ideas, different ways of living. If I encounter intolerance and ignorance, I try to be civilized in return. If someone turns hostile, I will leave him alone. I have seen too much pain and fought too many interior battles to engage in petty rhetoric or minor quarrels. I have never envied another man's worldly goods, because I realize that all the money in the world could not change my situation. I rejoice in the good health of relatives and friends, and strange as it may seem, have never wished to be in someone else's shoes.

So why do I get angry? My enemy is cunning, swift, powerful —and it strikes without warning. There is no way to counter the cruel movements of fate.

I am used to being attacked from within. I think of my circulatory system as a tangle of bureaucratic red tape; it has become so involved and complicated that it is out of my hands. I think of an insulin reaction as a red alert; everyone scrambles in panic, and no one will listen to reason.

But I don't think I will ever come to accept the random violence of the environment—a kind of violence I came to know.

After graduating from Boston University I moved to New York and rented an apartment in Queens. The building was a three-family brick house, and Freddy moved into the studio on the ground floor. The landlady was a middle-aged divorcee with bleached blond hair. She had the same kind of bitterness I have seen in many nurses over the years.

I settled in, looked for work during the day, and wrote short stories at night. I met an editor who said he wanted to publish a collection of my stories, so I worked on them every moment I could. Then the editor told me that he liked all the stories, but that they did not fit together. I was at a loss to understand. The volume was not published.

After a long search, I finally found a spot at Reader's Digest

Condensed Books as a reader. I would take home a suitcase full of books, read them, and make comments. I encountered hundreds of nubile governesses in search of true love on large estates; sexually agile spies fending off nuclear holocaust; jaded detectives; ax murderers; and bored, sex-starved housewives.

I read for about twelve hours a day, and then at night I wrote. Freddy came up often, but he was working six days a week as a plumber, going to school at night, and sleeping most of his free Sundays. I was alone most of the day in the house, and the only disturbance was the landlady screaming into the phone.

I asked her once, politely, if she could try to be a little quieter. She launched into an hour-long monologue on the sufferings of her life—and later moved furniture at two in the morning.

Every Tuesday I would go into Manhattan and pick up a new batch of books. I hated the idea of becoming a commuter; it wasn't the distance and time that bothered me, but the people. The rudeness of commuters is amazing, and the pace reminds me of the random collision of molecules.

On one such trip to the city, as I was emerging from the subway into the street a tiny sliver of steel struck my left eye and became embedded in the cornea. At the time I felt only a slight irritation, and rubbed my eyelid.

I almost lost my eye because of that random speck in space. I can never hope to make sense out of it: why that place, that time, me? An indiscriminate act of violence on the part of nature, another addition to a life of complications.

My eye, as Dr. Oculus later told me, began to rust.

I did not discover the sliver for three days. My eye became bloodshot and swollen, but I could find no reason for it. Then I looked in a mirror at an oblique angle and saw a tiny object shimmering in the light. I blinked—and suddenly it felt as though a sharp blade was cutting into the surface of my eye.

I went to the emergency room of a hospital, where I was asked if I had taken an overdose of drugs. I said I had taken half a dose, and that was why only one eye was bloodshot. Then I waited an hour, part of which I spent filling out forms—writing in large block letters that I was a diabetic.

They put me on a table next to a boy who had slit his wrists. Three doctors leaned over him, their white coats smeared with blood. The boy kept screaming that he wanted to die. He could not have been more than seventeen. I felt sorry for him: to be so young and have no reason to live. I thought of the many things I could never change, and it struck me that all my rebellion, all the destructive fighting against my body, was the product of an intense will to live. And at that moment, despite the pain and doubt and fright, I was happy that I at least had that desire.

A doctor came over, and I explained my problem. He shone a light in my eye. He could not see the speck.

I told him the object was lodged on the periphery of the cornea. I suggested that he examine my eye at an angle.

He found it, seeming as excited as an explorer. He didn't know what it was, but said he would try to lift it. He wrapped a wad of cotton around a long, thin stick and poked at the eye. It scraped the surface. The pain was a close second to the intensity of the needle in my foot. He told me the sliver was embedded too deeply, that I would have to see a specialist.

By now every time I blinked, the slicing pain returned, so the doctor taped a gauze pad over the eye.

I could no longer judge distance because I had lost my peripheral vision. I was afraid of having to move through the world this way for the rest of my life.

I didn't sleep that night.

Dr. Oculus agreed to see me the next morning in the hospital. He placed my head before a huge machine and looked for what seemed a long time.

"The eye is rusting," he said.

I did not understand.

He said that liquid and metal produce rust. He told me that he could remove the metal and some of the rust, but it was too deep to get it all out—he would run the risk of piercing the cornea.

I wished at that moment that I had been struck by a sliver of stainless steel. No such luck. Rusting! I thought of cars in junk yards.

The anger returned, the utter frustration of a life out of control. Each new twist was painful, defeating. And I fought back, because I did not want to end up on a hospital table with a river of blood flowing from my wrists.

Dr. Oculus put drops in my eye to deaden the nerves, then moved forward wielding a shiny scooplike instrument. I prayed that he might have steady hands. He touched my eye, and I moved, not out of pain, but revulsion.

He told me to stay still.

He scraped off the metal and the rusted cells of my cornea.

I asked if this condition would complicate my retinopathy.

He said it wouldn't help.

I wondered if I would be able to read with only one eye, and thought of what the world would be like for me without peripheral vision. Would I be knocked over by commuters on my blind side? I was angry, not at the doctor, but at my world of complications.

He told me to keep a patch on for a week, then to come back and he would examine the eye to see if the rusting was checked and the area healing.

I mentioned that every time I blinked I experienced an intense cutting pain.

He said the lid acted like a blade, slicing off the cells of my cornea; that was why the eye had to remain closed. He told me to rest as much as possible.

I went home, enraged at fate. My sugar rose, from anger and physical trauma. I tried to rest, but it was hard.

On the first of the month the landlady knocked on my door at seven in the morning and demanded the rent. I had always found a way to pay her on the first, and I said I would give her the rent later in the day but that I was sick and needed sleep.

She demanded it then.

I repeated that I would pay her later in the day. I said I had to rest or my eye would not heal. She stormed down and slammed her door. For the rest of the day that inventive woman made more noise than I thought possible for one human being. I thought the house was going to cave in. By midday she must have been exhausted, because the noise stopped and the stereo was turned up full blast.

I thought of my eye. I thought of my sugar. I knocked on her door and asked her please to be quiet, that my injured eye was a serious matter.

She said she didn't give a damn about my eye.

I told her I would not pay the rent if this situation continued. She screamed at me.

I walked back upstairs. It was impossible to sleep. I heard her screaming, and I figured she was on the phone because she paused at intervals. Suddenly the apartment was quiet. Just as I was losing consciousness, there was a knock on the door.

A policeman stood in the doorway. He was smiling. He said the woman downstairs had complained that I was a member of the Mafia and had threatened her life. I was also, according to the landlady, a pederast, thief, vandal, and junkie. She said I dressed in a police uniform and ran a protection racket.

I told the policeman that I had simply asked her for some peace and quiet because of my eye.

He said that he understood, that for my own peace of mind I should move.

The police returned nearly every day for various reasons: the landlady accused Freddy of being a flasher; said that I was throwing furniture down the stairs.

It was not the perfect environment for healing.

After an insane week, I returned to the doctor. Looking at the eye, he said the rust had not yet disappeared. He called over the nurse and asked if she wanted to see something unusual. She was interested in the rust, and the two of them talked about how I might lose the eye because of the spreading nature of the damage. I felt like an experimental animal, a specimen on the cutting table. They fell into an animated discussion of how rare it was to find a specimen with a rusty eye, and with retinopathy to boot. I wanted to scream: I am flesh and blood, don't you realize I am flesh and blood? I am afraid, I cannot sleep at night, and all I ask for is some comfort, or at least, common decency.

I wanted them to shut up just as I wanted the landlady to stop her senseless rantings. I wanted my eye to heal, but that was my concern. The world does not stop its course for the sick, the tired, the helpless. Nature can strike with a sliver of steel. And I must learn to keep my mouth shut, must learn not to complain because I can never change these things. I fight my own personal battles; I cannot fight fate.

But when I realize how insignificant I am in my powerlessness, I can begin to see all the wonders of life, appreciate the simple fact of seeing because it becomes more than just vision.

It becomes a gift—*a way of seeing*. My anger becomes tempered with simple joys. How marvelous it is to have a quiet landlady; to wake in the morning and see light filtering through the trees.

After several weeks, my eye healed. A scar remains, but my vision is not impaired. I moved to another apartment, and found quiet.

These simple facts seem to me miraculous, because for the rest of my life I will never forget that an eye can rust.

11

Till Death Do Us Part

WHEN I THINK of Carol I see her curled on a bed, her legs drawn close. I watch, and listen to the soft sound of her breathing as she sleeps. Her thick hair weaves and curls down her silken nape. Her hair is red, tendrils of flame across her face, and I find it odd that I am attracted to a color that reminds me of fire. Her legs are firm, slender; and in this sleeping position her spine is curved in a graceful arch. She moistens her lips, and I am enchanted by her unconscious movements. I think of how calm she is in sleep, and I am glad she can find peace.

I wake most nights at four in the morning, for no reason I know of. I get up and walk to the window. There is a dead stillness at that time, the silent hours of the morning. I am caught in the region between sleep and consciousness, and I feel a pressing, agitated force in my stomach, spreading to my feet. I seem to hear voices, the chattering of foreigners. Yet I understand them, all at the same time. They are trying to calm this angst in my soul, a terror welling up through my dreams that I cannot articulate. I walk around the apartment, listen to these conversations and take comfort.

When I am truly awake the voices run on, but I cannot understand a word. I always wake the second time in another room, and cannot remember how I got there. I sit for a long time and gaze at the empty street, and I feel a marvelous sense of peace. I stay awake, hoping I will not lose this feeling of security and comfort, but inevitably it begins to fade, and I check to make certain all the doors are bolted and the gas pilots are lit.

I think of Carol sleeping so peacefully on the bed. Carol, my wife, my love, guardian, and friend. I think of how far we have journeyed together, and my happiness and love are mixed with a tender sadness. I do not want her to suffer because of my fears, my pain. I want her to sleep and dream, and yet I cannot make any promises, cannot tell her that we will grow old together. I know how she worries about me, and I do not wake her because I also know she deserves the calm of sleep more than most people. She has to live with many restrictions and fears, all of them large and realistic. She lives in constant dread that I will have an insulin reaction on a New York subway and arms me with an arsenal of candy bars when I leave the house. She has endured the complications of my disease, has listened to the impersonal talk of doctors—and has had to sit back, knowing that there is nothing she can do, that all of her devotion cannot change things. A loved one's pain can be more acute than one's own; that is why I feel so strongly for Carol and my parents.

So at four in the morning I watch my wife sleeping, and know that her greatest fear is having to sleep alone. I do not want to leave her.

I met her the summer I was fifteen, the same year I met

Freddy and was beginning to let up on my withdrawal from life. It was a Wednesday night, when all the camp workers would meet at a bar to socialize. I was turned away from the door because I was too young. I borrowed proof of age from a lean six-footer of twenty-five, but it didn't work. I was only five foot eight. I tried again with the draft card of a 200-pounder, but I was more than fifty pounds lighter. I finally gave up, and my brother Ralph brought drinks out to me.

I was sitting there, leaning against a wall, when Carol walked over and asked if I was with the camp people. She said a friend of hers worked there. It turned out that we knew the same girl, and so we sat and talked.

We became friends that night. I was charmed by her exuberance, drawn by her open laughter and honesty. There was no sexual tension between us, nothing to prove.

It was the summer I discovered friendship. Freddy, two girls named Angie and Ginny, and Carol and I would all meet early on Saturday mornings and go to the beach. We sat in the sun and swam and talked, and the wind was like a tonic against my face.

I was learning to forget myself, but the diabetic mind does not stray for long. The symbol still returns twice a day: the needle. I do not view it as physical pain, because one becomes accustomed to that kind of discomfort. For me the insulin is the difference between life and death, the most crucial form of dependence. It can never be forgotten; it seeps through all relationships. When the juvenile diabetic matures to the point of understanding the concept of sharing, he is often stung by the realization that his loved ones will have to share his pain.

And a lover does not want to transfer pain; it can create both helplessness and guilt.

That summer when we became friends, Carol almost lost her

life. It was a humid day in July, and we were at the beach. The lifeguards were on strike. I had swum to a sandbar about two hundred yards out. When I came back, the undertow was strong and the swim to shore exhausted me.

I was wading in the shallow water when Ralph, Freddy, Ginny, and Carol decided they would swim to the sandbar. I told them about the undertow and warned them against going. They swam off.

Swimming back to shore, Carol panicked. Ralph and Freddy tried to hold her up, but she fought them and went down. By the time Ralph and Freddy pulled her up again, she was unconscious. Together they towed her back to shore.

Unaware of any of this, I suddenly saw a crowd gather on the beach. Then through the crowd I glimpsed a long lock of red hair matted with sand. I ran and pushed through; a state trooper was holding an oxygen mask over her face. I tried to see if her chest was moving.

Her eyes opened, and then she struggled to her feet—only to fall flat on her back. They took her away in an ambulance, and I waited on the sand for more than an hour, thinking that perhaps she was dead. I was reminded of my grandfather and my cousin, of the flame from a liturgical candle . . .

Carol recovered, but from that day on I was afraid of love, afraid of sharing my life. There was the possibility of pain in my future, and I did not want to impose my suffering on another person. The *possibility* of complications, of an early death, always intruded on my thoughts of a future, especially one shared with another person. I do not buy the attitude that "it could happen to anyone." What counts is that the diabetic lives with the potential of crisis every day of his life, and it is his responsibility to come to terms with the possibilities if he is to become involved with another person.

After we had been good friends for three years, Carol came to visit me in Boston. She told me she was in love with me. I could not answer her. I did not think she understood the kind of commitment that would be necessary, the severity and swiftness of change in my personal life. I felt sad because she was offering me a gift, and I could not reach out and take it naturally, easily. I wanted to love and share without fear. It could never be that easy.

For a long time, I would not say I loved her, but Carol is a crafty woman, and I underestimated her resolve. I tried to discourage her, told her of all the frightening possibilities ahead of me. She listened and understood and told me she did not care.

And so that night I told Carol I loved her, because I was tired of solitude and truly wanted to share my life. I yearned to give to another person; I had lived too long with myself. And I thought that Carol was right, that we could share an intense love, perhaps for a few years, perhaps longer.

I refused to marry, though, for over four years. The capacity to love was one thing, but marriage seemed an awesome step, entailing the kind of responsibility that I could not guarantee. I thought it would be easier for Carol to cope with illness or death if we were not married. If I went blind it would present countless demands on her, and I did not want her to feel burdened. I would rather have had her leave and remember me well than cater to an impossible invalid. Marriage seemed cruel.

But she was already involved, and there was nothing I could do to kill her emotions. I really did not want to lose her, because her love seemed a purification, an easing of pain. And if I lived with the fear of hurting Carol, I also learned the immense joy of forgetting myself in the goodness of another person.

I was caught, and the road became painful.

She learned many things, gripping my arm while we sat in waiting rooms, and it was frustrating to watch the fears grow in her mind, because there was no way I could comfort her. She learned to fear blindness, infections, gangrene, insulin reactions, coma, arteriosclerosis, strokes, kidney damage, heart attacks, death. I could easily leave her with nothing, and I began to live with a sense of guilt and betrayal. But she would not give up, and I will always thank her for the depth of her commitment.

Before we were married, Carol came to me one day and said she had talked to both a priest and a doctor, and that both had recommended that she run as far away from me as possible. They said that I would not live very long, that I was selfish to involve Carol in my life. The doctor said that I would become impotent (a subject I'll take up in the next chapter), that if we did have children before that event they would become diabetic, that I would become a hopeless invalid and then leave her a young widow. The priest also said that I would lose my sexual vigor, and seconded all the doctor's other notions.

I was jolted and angry. Their questioning may have been valid, but there was an important factor that neither of these men bothered to consider, and that was why their smug advice enraged me: *they did not know me, had never seen me or talked with me; we were complete strangers.* In my view, that single fact made them incapable of judgment. My capacity for love and goodness was never considered by either man.

Does the duration of a relationship reflect its quality? Would the priest have advised the apostles to run from Christ because they would only know him for three years? Would the knowledge of inevitable crucifixion have changed their relationship?

Whether the priest and doctor spoke from knowledge, much of what they said could prove true. But surely love is not invalidated by illness. The fact that my love could cause great pain did not make it selfish. Perhaps love becomes more valuable when each moment is so important.

The capacity and intensity of love must be weighed in the present. The future is a consideration to be questioned; and a balance, an understanding, must be reached from within, not by outsiders.

I weighed those questions.

How could I marry Carol with the possibility of so much illness in the future? There is a horror more frightening than actual blindness: I have seen it in waiting rooms, in hospitals, on the street. It is the involvement of the person who has been drawn into the sphere of illness because of a special relationship.

It is a peculiar type of anger and hatred, born out of love and a sense of loss. The world changes, more than just physically. One lover becomes a frightened child, moving in a world of darkness. The other becomes a mother. The blind one often whimpers, loses his strength, becomes dependent. He wants constant attention, and the other begins to resent his hanging on. Rage builds within each of them: the blind one angered at his visual loss, his incapacitation; the other feeling like a nursemaid, a slave. The sense of sharing is lost. The universe of love becomes distorted by anger.

I have seen that kind of anger, and I fear it. I do not want Carol to spend her life leading me by the arm. I am afraid that my anger against my body would turn against her, my frustration become a weapon. If I lose my eyes, she will lose her independence. That is a high price. It is not a matter of her dedication; I am not afraid that she will leave me. I often think that might be easier.

But my chances of going blind are twenty-five times greater

than those of a nondiabetic. And I have no way of knowing how either of us will react.

Statistics on the diabetic's life span differ, but none of the figures is comforting. The disease is expensive, and I do not want to leave a poor widow. Diabetics, especially juveniles, are often turned down for life insurance.

Then there is the question of children. The implications of heredity are enormous. Research on the role played by heredity in the disease is ongoing, and much still remains to be learned. When a diabetic marries a nondiabetic who is not a carrier, the probability is that none of the children will become diabetic, but they will all be carriers. If two carriers marry, 25 percent of the offspring will become diabetic, 75 percent carriers. For a diabetic and a carrier, the ratio is 50 percent diabetic, 50 percent carriers. And *all* the children of two diabetics will contract the disease eventually. It should be noted, though, that there are exceptions to all these rules.

There are 10 million diabetics in this country today—and perhaps as many as 10 million others who are undiagnosed. *And there are more than 50 million carriers,* 50 million time bombs hidden in the population. The number of diabetics will double every fifteen years. The average American born today has a better than one in five chance of developing diabetes. We are spreading a disease for which there is no cure.

In the face of all these questions, the price of love becomes steep. But Carol and I married. We have been happy for each day we have had together.

And now I watch her stomach swell with our first child. I am awed by this miracle, feel a sense of warmth I have never known when I think of the baby. I am also concerned, as every parent, for a normal birth.

There are those who would say that I have no right to bring

children into this world. It has not been an easy decision. Carol and I discussed the matter for over two years. We finally decided that we wanted to share our lives with children: our entire lives. We knew, more than most, that sharing also includes the possibility of great pain in the future.

I will pass down, among other traits, diabetes. That fact will haunt me for the rest of my life.

A person cannot pass down anything more valuable than love, and I will love my child forever.

I look at Carol in the early morning when I wake, and I pray that she will not suffer. I ask the Creator to give me time, and I am thankful for what we have been able to share.

But there are times when I am afraid because I do not want to leave her.

12

Extremities

MOST DIABETICS SUFFER from neuropathy, simply defined as any disease of the nervous system. Peripheral nerves are those lining the brain and spinal cord, and they are the source of diabetic malfunctions of the extremities. Often several feet long, the peripheral nerves are covered by a membrane, and for some reason associated with diabetes, the walls of the membrane thicken and nerve function is impaired because conduction of impulses is slowed.

All diabetics suffer from some alteration of these nerves, which can cause severe pain. The National Commission on Diabetes reported: "One half of these symptoms are severe enough to cause partial or total disability, accompanied by intense pain and eventual loss of sensation. The anesthetized extremities are susceptible to injury and ulceration, which may contribute, in many cases, to the loss of the affected extremity."

The report went on to say that fewer than six researchers worldwide were looking into the problems of neuropathy.

Because virtually every organ of the body can be ravaged by diabetic complications, there is believed to be some connection between the small blood vessels that feed the nerves and the destruction of the nerve membrane.

I have no real explanation for the pain in my legs, can only hope for the easing that occasionally takes place. The pain has become another fact of life, one I try to ignore. Accepting the pain in my legs, I can put it aside and get on with the business of living. I will not spend my life living with dreams of a cure, nor will I sit on my bed and summon angels. I would rather walk down the street and feel the warmth of the sun against my face, pain in my legs or not. There is a balance, and perhaps I have learned to appreciate that feeling of warmth more than most people. If I cannot change my condition, at least I can alter my way of seeing things. Complaining changes nothing. I very rarely mention that I am in pain. I have no need of sympathy. I try to keep my fears in the back of my mind; I need a sense of proportion about myself. Whatever I have suffered, I have also been given many gifts: I have survived, and I possess the will to continue to survive.

There is another extremity—the center of both great pleasure and intense anxiety—that is often damaged by neuropathy. Diabetes is a major cause of impotence, one of the rare physical causes of sexual dysfunction.

The prospect frightens me as much or more than any other complication. The figures vary; estimates run as high as 80 percent, but the most common statistic is that about 50 percent of diabetic males become impotent. Doctors tend to ignore this possibility, and I understand why. There is nothing they can do, and the psychological implications for the patient, if he is aware of the problem, can be overwhelming.

I first learned of it by accident. I was reading one of those pop-psychology how-to articles in a popular women's magazine —a guide to handling an impotent lover. After a lot of make-him-feel-like-a-man-and-let-him-know-he's-a-bedroom-acrobat advice, I came across this parenthetical sentence: "Diabetes is one of the few physical causes for impotence." There was no other mention of the problem as it related to diabetes.

I felt the old sense of powerlessness returning. Still another thing in life I would not be able to control.

Naturally, I began to investigate further. I learned that erectile tissue is made up of a spongelike system of blood lakes between arteries and veins. Erection occurs when these spaces are filled with blood; in order for this to happen, the penile arteries have to dilate. The response is controlled by the nerves. Neuropathy causes beaded thickening and damage to the nerves, making dilation of the arteries, and therefore erection, impossible. (Autopsies performed on five diabetic males in Argentina in 1974 showed marked damage of neurologic origin in four of the men. The severity and duration of diabetes had proved to be major factors in the onset of impotence. At the same time, no degree of damage to the penile tissues was found in a control group of five nondiabetic males.)

Sexual activity takes place in four stages: libido, erection, orgasm, and ejaculation. Quite often, diabetic impotence affects only the erection response. And so I am afraid of living, some day, in a perpetual state of horniness.

The libido is the erotic zone of the psyche, which supplies the initial spark of human sexuality. The mind is the most stimulating organ of the body. We create images, and they in turn

provoke carnal responses. Once the penis fills with blood and
becomes erect, orgasm and ejaculation can follow.

Imagine the frustration for an impotent diabetic: his libido is
intact, his imagination strong. *He is excited—in his mind he is
excited.* But his penis will not respond. The desire for sexual
stimulation is present; the mechanism is lost. How can he find
satisfaction?

Technicalities aside, there remains the psychological problem of lost manhood. This actually seems to me a silly concern.
We have somehow made sex the focal point of the male universe. But I do not sit and contemplate my manhood; I consider
my humanity. My member is mindless. It proves nothing to me
beyond its simple physical ability to engorge with blood. I, as
a human being, have to stand tall; not just my penis.

It would be foolish to say that I would not suffer if I did
develop diabetic impotence. But I do not think I would question
my manhood. To survive, to retain some measure of human
kindness and compassion, to be capable of love in the face of
pain and setbacks—these are the qualities of manhood. To
accept great loss and sorrow, to deal with questions that can
never be resolved, to concentrate on my abilities and gifts—this
is the humanity I strive toward. I would rather lose the use of
my mindless penis than any of these qualities.

If I become impotent, I hope I can adjust to the loss. For me,
I think it would most truly be felt in the loss of intimacy.

With someone else to consider, the loss of physical love
becomes painful. I do not have to prove to Carol that I am a
man; we do not view sexual love as a performance. But the loss
would be painful because of the bond of sharing that we feel
when making love. It is a symbol of commitment and a culmi-
nation of emotions. It causes me to forget completely the other
physical matters that complicate my life—and how ironic that

it is another possible source of pain related to diabetes. There are other ways to relieve sexual tension, but there is no way to replace the sense of closeness.

We respond to the question of impotence by accepting the possibility—and sharing intensely the sexual joys of the present. If the loss occurs, I only hope I am man enough to deal with it.

13

Degeneration

I HAVE SPENT MOST of my life struggling to understand. I have grown up with frustration and anger, physically and psychologically scarred from the age of ten. I can never forget that frightened child.

Every diabetic reaction triggers a memory shooting back to the onset of illness. I see the child, unable to comprehend the physical changes. He performs blind rituals of medical faith, but his new religion offers no comfort, only tends to reinforce a sense of alienation. He follows dogma with childlike faith, but his obedience is not rewarded by either healing or peace. He is ravaged by the brittle fluctuations in blood sugar; both ends of the spectrum produce extreme reactions.

As the young diabetic grows, he can either try to deny the existence of his disease or search for knowledge. Ignorance only causes further damage; darkness can only produce unfounded fears. The diabetic cannot hide; he can merely try to ignore. But his body will remind him.

Denial also results in ignorance, which means excluding many helpful aspects of care. In this era of specialized medicine, the diabetic must choose the caretakers of his body with caution. *The diabetic, in fact, needs to know more than his doctor.*

A podiatrist is ignorant of the complications of diabetic feet. He has no knowledge of the *scope* of the problem. Most specialists don't.

It is therefore my responsibility, as a diabetic, to know the medical aspects of my condition, to be informed to the point where I myself am capable of judgment. I must be aware of the total picture, because I live in a world of specialists. I must be able to inform them of possible complications.

Unfortunately, some doctors, like other men, cannot, or will not, admit to ignorance. And like other men, they make mistakes, or simply do not care.

The diabetic's responsibility to himself is enormous. The issue, for him, is nothing less than survival. Knowledge is his only weapon.

Knowledge can be hard to handle.

When the diabetic is aware of the nature of his disease, the future can get clouded indeed. But we must know—for our own physical good, and for the benefit of those we are involved with.

Diabetes filters through and alters every aspect of a life, and that single fact makes it crucial for the diabetic to understand his disease. It would have been immoral of me to marry Carol if she were not fully aware of diabetic realities: from impotence to the prospect of an early death. I could not tell her for certain if any of these things would happen; no one knows. But intimate involvement is rooted in honesty and a sense of responsibility.

Those we love are directly affected by the disease. They need to know the price of commitment.

If I am to function, I must form a relationship with the disease itself. As I have matured, I have felt a great need to lay the ghosts of past irrational fears to rest. It seems to me now that this yearning is nothing less than the quest for identity, for the disease is inseparable from life.

My fear of the unknown was centered within my body, and I lived with the premonition of a coming explosion. Mystery produces unrelieved tension. That is no way to live.

So I searched for the facts. And they turned out to be just as frightening as the anxieties. Each new revelation seemed a slap in the face, another setback in the struggle.

As I gathered the statistics, I tried to keep in mind that they were not rules. I realize the possibility that I might be an exception, that I might be spared some of the complications. But I must also accept the fact that I have a good chance of becoming one of the numbers. I will not know until the time comes.

I have come to hate the statistics. I stare at the numbers, wishing I could change them. But I must realize that fifteen years of the more serious juvenile form have already produced irreversible damage. I do not want to leave this world too soon. But . . .

Three hundred thousand diabetics die every year.

The number will rise with the annual 6 percent increase in the number of diabetics. Death is usually the slow and painful result of complications. The National Commission on Diabetes reports that 14 percent of the diabetic population is bedridden for an average of forty-five days a year. No other chronic disease is so incapacitating.

Most of the diabetic complications are rooted in the vascular system. For a reason scientists don't yet fully understand, the circulatory system becomes clogged with metabolic debris. Virtually every organ of the body is affected. And organs are slowly destroyed.

Blindness is a terrible burden, not a killer. But the diabetic suffering from retinopathy has a debris-strewn vascular system that is the cause of his blindness. He will therefore suffer from more lethal problems related to circulatory impairment.

Diabetics are seventeen times more likely to suffer from kidney disease than nondiabetics. The process is identical to the spread of retinopathy. Tufts of capillaries form a complex network in the kidneys, carrying blood so that the cells can filter waste products and provide oxygen. The same thickening of cell membranes occurs in the kidneys as in the eyes.

Man cannot live if his kidneys do not work. Nearly 100 percent of all diabetics suffer from impaired kidney function, and 50 percent of all juvenile diabetics die from kidney failure. Dialysis has proved to be a help in buying time, but it is not a cure.

Diabetics are five times more likely to get gangrene than nondiabetics. Again, it is a problem of circulation: the blood cannot filter waste products. Infection leads to gangrene, and gangrene leads to amputation.

A clogged vascular system is the curse of diabetes: Arteriosclerosis, a usual part of the aging process, is greatly accelerated in the diabetic. The risk of heart attack is estimated at two to five times higher in the diabetic. Strokes occur five times more often in the diabetic than in the nondiabetic.

I was not very surprised when I saw the figures on life span. The average length of life after onset of diabetes, I have read, is 18.1 years. The figures vary: the highest I've seen is a reduction of the average life expectancy by one-third.

Not bad if you become a diabetic at the age of fifty. Not bad when you consider that the life span of a diabetic in 1914 was 4.9 years after onset.

But I became a diabetic at the age of ten.

We cannot live with statistics. In three years I will have had diabetes for eighteen years. I will not then act as if I have 0.1 year to live. Aware of the severity of my disease, I try to control my blood sugar. There is even a medical faction that contends that control is not important. They cite cases of strictly controlled diabetics who have suffered severe complications. But the diabetic process remains a mystery, and such a conclusion as yet has no scientific basis. Since we know that high blood sugar kills, it seems reasonable to try to maintain a blood-sugar level that is close to the norm.

Money is needed for an intensive effort to wipe out these statistics of death. We can only hope that the public will become aware of the problem before they become intimately involved with the disease. The National Commission on Diabetes report was responsible for additional government funding for research, but much more is needed.

To achieve this, diabetics must band together to exert pressure; even if it is too late for them, they might save their children. The Juvenile Diabetes Foundation, founded in 1972, has done a great deal to foster the necessary awareness of the disease and to raise funds for research. Unfortunately, the public only seems to become involved when it is touched or frightened by the problem. In this respect, ironically, the high incidence of diabetes is an advantage. Seventy million people in this country should be touched or frightened: diabetics; their relatives who are carriers; and those who are susceptible—the obese, the aged, and those with poor nutritional habits. These people will suffer, and they will die in great numbers.

If the figures are not sobering enough, consider this single sentence tucked within the National Commission report: "With an increasing population and an escalating incidence of diabetes, there is serious concern that adequate supplies of insulin will no longer be available from animal pancreases." Animals are the only source of insulin we have at present. (Genetic experiments have produced human insulin in bacterial cultures, but production is a long way off.) Diabetics cannot live without it; you cannot ration insulin.

We are kept alive by the good grace of pigs and cows. Insulin is not a cure, but it is the only means we have of fighting diabetes at the present time. It sustains life, buys time. Before the discovery of insulin, diabetics died within a few years of onset, and those with the juvenile form did not stand a chance. As the disease spreads and the supply of insulin dwindles, we face a future in which decisions may have to be made about who will live and who will die.

I will pass down the diabetic gene. I am horrified by the possibility that my children, or my children's children, might not have even the time that insulin supplies.

The only hope for the future is awareness of the facts. I set out to find some answers, to plan for the future and learn to live with the painful possibilities. I feel some measure of peace because I have told the truth to those I love. I can live with fear; I cannot live with lies.

Will I become a blind, impotent amputee with heart disease who is carried to the dialysis center three times a week? Will I die prematurely?

All of the above?

Some of the above?

None of the above?

I have no way of knowing. I can only live through whatever time I have, trying to beat the numbers. Trying to live productively.

And every day, I will pray for future generations.

14

Backups

I AM PROUD of my style—one-handed, blind—when I inject insulin into my buttocks.

A shot in the ass. My form and delivery are perfection, refined to an art over the years. I clean the vials and twist off the plastic covers on the disposable syringe. I suck the insulin into the tube with a quick motion, then push back to expel air bubbles.

It is a ritual developed over fifteen years. When I wake in the morning I pace the floor for several minutes, trying to clear my head before I get to the needle. I know from experience that if I am not fully awake, later on I may not be sure whether I have taken the injection.

I perform the rite in the kitchen. I like to sit near a window, where the sun streams through. I always open the shades because I feel comforted by the morning light. I take great pleasure just in looking, in being able to see.

When I am ready, I drop my pants. Standing, I rub the soft flesh with cleansing alcohol. The coldness of the liquid is uncomfortable in the winter, and quite pleasant in the warmer months. Should I move south for the winter?

I take the needle in my hand and twist my arm backward, turning my palm so that the needle is pointed toward my flesh. I turn my head but cannot see where I'll be injecting. I keep my eyes on the needle, moving my arm in a slow, rhythmic pattern, trying to keep my hand trained on the vicinity of impact—the area of skin that is tingling from the coolness of the alcohol.

As always, I hesitate. My way of life, and my destiny, health, the way I think, my fears, have been tied to this ritual for so many years. The relationship will exist for the rest of my life.

On impact, I feel the skin cave in and a tinge of pain. Without seeing, I press the needle in until I feel the base of the syringe come in contact with the skin. I slide my middle finger along the underside of the syringe, trying to balance the mass of plastic and steel protruding from my posterior. When I reach the plunger, still balancing the syringe with my middle finger, I curve my thumb and push. The nectar of life oozes into my body.

I pull the needle out and swab the area with alcohol. The cotton pad I use for swabbing is often covered with blood. That is the only result I see of the whole operation.

When Carol and I were first married we took a ground-floor apartment. The windows were at eye level, and I must have gained a reputation as both a flasher and a junkie during the year we lived there—although I should mention that anyone looking in the window would have to crane his neck and look down at an angle. He'd have to go out of his way to see in.

One spring morning, after watching birds gather near the windows, I horrified an old woman passing by. Her hair was white, pulled back in a tight bun, and her stockings were rolled around her ankles. Not more than fifteen feet away, she saw my twisted body the needle, the bare ass. I saw her mouth open. She would not move on. I felt the need to explain because I saw the look on her face. A perverted junkie, she was saying to herself. I wanted to tell her that this needle represented life for me, not death.

But I understood that there was no way to explain; people do not want to listen. I was once detained on the American side of the Canadian border because the customs officials refused to believe that I was a diabetic. They tore apart my car in search of illicit drugs, and refused to let me go to the bathroom until the search was finished. People believe what they want to. Ever since that incident, I have carried a doctor's note when traveling. As the customs official said: anyone can buy insulin and a medical alert tag. The world is paranoid.

Later that spring day, I saw the old woman outside again, pointing at my window. A police officer stood next to her. He did not bother to come in and arrest me. But from that time on, I closed the shades. It angered me at the time, though I can look back and joke about it now. There is no reason why others should be subjected to my seemingly freakish behavior.

My anger then had little connection with diabetes, though there are many emotions directly related to the diabetic condition. It is well known that changes in blood chemistry can alter moods. The anger I experience during an insulin reaction is actually a result of the physical changes taking place within my body. Depression, too, is a symptom of diabetes, also attributable to the chemical changes of the diabetic process.

The answer, of course, is to try to keep the blood-sugar level as close to the norm as possible. The diabetic must realize that these feelings will leave when control is maintained. The condition is not permanent. It is comforting to know the reason for these feelings, to understand that when depression or anger strikes for no reason, I am not losing my mind.

If blood-sugar levels and chemical changes can alter emotions, it is also true that emotions can alter sugar levels and chemical balances.

When I get angry because of outside forces not connected with diabetes, my sugar rises. *Always.* There are also physical changes: my mouth gets dry, and I will spend the night going to and from the bathroom. The urine flows in a long, slow stream. I will test it, and find an excess of sugar spilling from my kidneys. My eyes will go out of focus. The weakness spreads through my body. I begin to dehydrate, and have to consume large amounts of water to quench my thirst.

These are chemical, not psychological, changes. How does the diabetic handle emotional alterations of his physical condition? I am talking about some of the ordinary frustrations of everyday living, which can make a diabetic physically ill. I cannot, and would not want to suppress my emotions all the time. Valium is not the answer, only a crutch. We must learn to deal with our passions, conquer them and get on with the business of living.

It is not always easy.

Which brings me back to that ground-floor apartment. The old woman was a minor source of anger, easy enough to forget. But another event over which I had no control kept my anger, and my sugar, high for weeks.

The apartment was always damp because the water pipes for the entire building were located under our floor. House plants thrived in the tropical climate; in fact moss was beginning to grow in the closets and along the walls. But while our plants flourished, I did not; the dampness caused a great deal of discomfort, especially in my legs. The building superintendent speculated about the possibility of a break in one of the pipes as the cause of the excessive dampness.

On a moist September night, Carol woke me at two A.M. to listen to a strange sound.

It was water gurgling.

I went into the bathroom and saw water bubbling in the toilet bowl. Carol was afraid the water would overflow; I told her not to worry and to go back to sleep.

She woke me again at four. The gurgling had not stopped, and the water was rising in the bowl. She had not gone back to sleep, but had spent two hours leaving messages on the tape machine in the super's office.

She had then gone ahead and called a sewer company. A man told her that what we'd seen and heard meant that pipes in the building were backed up, and there would be tremendous problems if things were not fixed before people started getting up in the morning. There were sixty apartments in the building.

My friend Freddy is a plumber, and I am always amazed by the exotic things he tells me he finds in people's drains and pipes. I didn't want to see intimate details of my neighbors' lives flowing through my halls. But the sewer man had told Carol he couldn't do anything about the problem unless he was authorized by the management of the building—and we couldn't reach the super, though he allegedly carried one of those beepers that doctors use.

By five in the morning the toilet started to overflow. Human waste and the flotsam of private lives began to rise from the drain in the shower. By six the pressure was so high that the grill popped off the shower drain.

Carol began to panic. She moved all the clothes from the

closet to the bed. The smell was sickening. The cat ran for high ground and seemed amused. I closed the bathroom door to try to contain the flood.

Water, feces, and debris spilled from under the door and into the closet. People in the building were beginning to get up, and their waste poured into our apartment with great force. The rug in the bedroom was covered, and excrement clung to the legs of the bed. Carol wanted me to do something. I told her I could not part the Red Sea.

By seven the waste was floating down the hallway as I went outside and waited by the maintenance office. Forty minutes later I was able to tell one of the handymen about the problem. He said they would take care of it right away.

At that time I was working in Manhattan for a paperback publishing house. Carol didn't want me to leave, but I felt I had to go to the office because I had taken the previous day off to visit the eye doctor. I assured her they would stop the flood within the hour.

Poor Carol. I should have stayed home. No one came to fix the pipes. The super told Carol that he needed authorization from the management. Carol called the office every fifteen minutes. The secretary refused to let her speak to the building agent.

She called me every hour to keep me informed of the water level; it went over a foot high.

The secretary at the main office told Carol every time she called that they were sending repairmen. They had known of the problem for four hours, and still no one came. At noon, the secretary hung up while Carol was begging her to send help. Much of our furniture was already ruined.

I called the main office at one in the afternoon. I was angry, and my sugar was high. I couldn't remember if I had taken my insulin during the confusion of the morning. Carol had been crying most of the day.

I told the secretary my name and asked to speak to the manager. She told me that my wife had been calling all morning.

I asked again to speak to the manager.

She said that they were sending someone over to fix the pipes.

I told her that someone should have dealt with the problem five hours before.

"Don't get nasty," she said.

I said that she did not seem to understand the problem, and asked again for the manager.

She demanded to know what kind of problem—then she would decide if I could speak to the manager.

"The problem," I said, "is that I have a foot of water and shit floating through my apartment." I was disgusted with the bureaucratic tangle.

"Don't you use foul language with me," she said.

"You don't seem to understand," I said. "Shit is literally floating through my apartment."

"I will not stand for filthy talk," she said.

"You want me to call it excrement, lady? You want me to call it feces? It comes down to the same thing."

"You just watch your tongue," she said.

She didn't care a bit, I realized, about what was floating through our home. It was not her problem; she was safe and dry in her high-rise office.

"You really couldn't give a damn, could you," I said.

"That's right."

I said then that I would have to make it her problem. I told her that if the sewage pouring into my apartment was not stopped immediately I would come down to her office and sling a bag of shit in her face. I said that might help her understand what we were going through.

She gasped.

"Excuse me," I said. "Make that excrement. I'll sling a bag of excrement in your face."

She hung up.

They stopped the flood waters at three in the afternoon and sent a man down to mop the floors. One reason we had taken the apartment was that Carol loved the parquet floors. The water had made them buckle and separate. Waste material was wedged between the spaces.

We couldn't sleep in the apartment that night because of the odor. There were water marks and excrement stains on the walls. A professional cleaner came the next day and said that dangerous bacteria had seeped under the floor, and the apartment would not be safe until the flooring was ripped out, the base cleaned, and the wood replaced. The manager refused to replace the flooring; nor did he offer to pay for the damage to the furniture. (The owners of the building paid us damages later on in a settlement, after we had sued.)

We left the apartment immediately, and depended on the kindness of relatives for shelter for the next month. We had to go to the doctor for shots against the bacteria we had been exposed to.

My sugar remained high for weeks. I had been powerless for over eight hours, at the mercy of people who did not care about my problems. I had to sit back and watch what I had worked for being destroyed literally by other people's shit. The realization that I could have been helped if others had merely shown some consideration heightened my frustration. There had been no reason for them to stall us for so long. It's the kind of problem urban dwellers face all the time, but it had a special effect on me.

I fought to bring my sugar to a reasonable level, which in the end is all a diabetic can do. But I realized that to control my disease I must learn certain attitudes that are healthy for any human being. I try to ignore the petty matters that so often anger people. I will not waste my time and raise my sugar in useless battles. I do not fight with people who have different opinions. I would not argue if someone told me the moon was square.

Most important, I have learned to forget. I refuse to dwell on my past frustrations. I have learned the value of a sense of humor, of being able to see things in perspective. My first obligation is to control my sugar. If I hold on to hate and anger I will become physically sick.

15

Unanswered Questions

A LONG TIME AGO I picked up a book on diabetes that was written just after the discovery of insulin in 1921. Doctors then were beginning to learn of the complications of diabetes because patients were surviving longer with the help of insulin. The book told me that it was highly likely that death would be caused by blood-vessel disease—heart attack, stroke, kidney failure.

I took diabetic death to mean my death.

The author went on to say that I should be "reassured" that it was highly likely that I would live "at least" until my thirties, and that there was a 1-in-27 chance of my surviving into my forties.

The volume is dated now, of course; the numbers have changed over the years. But the attitude, in many respects, has remained the same.

I am not comforted by the fact that my survival stock has

risen a few points. I understand that doctors are delighted and proud of lengthening life spans. But the progress is slow in the search for a cure. And they deal with the disease in such a detached manner. I have no quarrel with the scientific method; objectivity is a valuable tool in many ways, probably the only way to proceed in the quest for a solution. But it is my life that is hanging in the balance.

And I am not reassured by the prospect of living a few more years. The simple fact that the number has risen is not comforting to someone who falls within the range of those numbers. An unemployment figure of only 5 percent is not very comforting to a person out of work.

In a recent book called *Diabetes Explained: A Layman's Guide,* written by Dr. Ira J. Laufer and Herbert Kadison (Saturday Review Press, 1976), the authors state that the diabetic can expect to live in a fashion "closely approaching the normal." They go on to state that the life expectancy after onset of diabetes rose to 18.1 years in 1970, and that it is no doubt higher at present.

That might be a nice figure, but not for someone who was stricken at the age of ten. Doctors forget we are humans, not numbers, and it is hard to excuse that unintentional callousness. I think of the painful journey to acceptance and become angered by such statements. They show an ignorance of the diabetic's true concern: how to live as productively as possible in the time one has. They also seem oblivous to the problem of how to handle the psychological fears connected with the disease.

On the subject of impotence, the same book tells me that intercourse is not the only way to satisfy the sexual urge. The authors mention manual and oral sex as a substitute for genital-to-genital contact.

They miss the whole point. I am not a robot. I am a man in love, and I am not concerned with the mechanical aspects of lovemaking. I am not concerned with screwing but with sharing. I fear the loss of intimacy. I fear the possible tension created by the loss of an important form of expression.

I think of my wife crying at night because she is afraid she will be alone. I think of the terrible weight I have placed on the shoulders of those I love. Nowhere do the authors mention the price of commitment.

I look at my father, who would give me almost anything in the world I wanted. But he cannot give me health. I see, at times, that he would give everything he has if he could cure me. That is the highest measure of love, and I carry a great deal of guilt because of the possibility that I might die before him, and cannot repay his concern.

I have seen my mother, too, and my brothers and sister become sick with fear over the years. I have kept my mouth shut in the hope of sparing them pain.

No one seems to have bothered to write about problems like these. Diabetics and their families are human, and that is the most serious complication of the disease. We live with a great deal of pressure, and the only way to release it is to discuss these concerns.

The Laufer and Kadison book is instructive for the diabetic and the nondiabetic who know little about the disease. I myself do not find the pep-talk sections very helpful.

I have read many books dealing with diabetes, all of them written by doctors. Without exception, the literature fails to deal with the emotional concerns and fears of the diabetic. The few books I mention here are, for me, representative of the literature in general and have had the most impact personally.

There is another book that bothers me a great deal: *Diabetes:*

New Look at an Old Problem (Harper & Row, 1976). This book, too, might be helpful for those who are ignorant of the medical aspects of the disease. The authors, Dr. Bertrand E. Lowenstein and Paul D. Preger, Jr., devote considerable space to discussion of symptoms and complications. Their tone, however, reminds me of the rest of the maddening literature. One example is their insistence that a juvenile is not a diabetic, but a child with diabetes. I am sure their intentions are good, but I find the statement condescending.

I was not a stupid child. You do not keep telling a child he can lead a normal life if he is normal. It is the surest sign that something is wrong and he really isn't normal. I spent much of my young life trying to deny the fact that I was a diabetic. I feel no shame now in calling myself one. My life has been changed by the disease, and to deny that is to admit to some kind of shame.

In discussing retinopathy, Lowenstein and Preger say that 40 percent of all diabetics develop problems to some degree, and that another 40 percent develop serious problems and "face trouble." They go on to say that the diabetic should not *assume* he will be in that group.

That is very easy to say. But try living with the possibility of blindness. I can assume nothing, and that has been one of the main problems in my life. Forty percent is a number *I* have to live with, not the doctors. I assume nothing, because I don't know very much for certain. But I must prepare myself for possibilities because my life and the lives of those around me will be changed if I go blind. I wouldn't want to deal with those questions the day *after* I lose my sight.

But there is a far more serious disservice rendered by this book. The authors state as their opinion that insulin is the cause of the vascular complications of diabetes. Insulin produced by the nondiabetic normally travels from the pancreas directly to the liver, where it is stored, used, and distributed throughout the body. As a result, very little is present in the bloodstream at any given time. But injections of insulin travel in large concentrations through the bloodstream first, and then to the liver. The authors speculate that this concentration of insulin in the bloodstream causes vascular complications.

They go on to say that no diabetic should be taking more than 30 to 40 units of insulin per day, citing an insurance company study that stated that diabetics taking more than 30 units of insulin had a death rate more than six times the norm. I have taken over 70 units of insulin in a day, during my growing years, and I am now stable at just over 40 units per day.

A few weeks after reading this particular book, I found that my sugar was out of control; I was ill with the symptoms of high blood sugar. I found I had unthinkingly lowered my insulin dose. I also found that I cannot live on the amount of insulin the authors prescribe.

Theirs is dangerous speculation because the complications of the disease remain a mystery. To tell a diabetic that he might suffer blindness, amputation, kidney disease, or death because of his insulin leaves him very little in the way of choices. The authors cannot know the severity of the reader's condition. They do mention that the reader should consult his doctor, but their theory could affect a diabetic mind already filled with fears.

The mind reacts in strange ways. I did not know I was lowering my insulin dose. The Lowenstein/Preger theory might be interesting, but there are no conclusive results. No one knows what causes the complications of diabetes.. The potential danger of insulin is another fear I must come to accept, but I cannot stop taking it.

The authors seem not to have realized the psychological impact of revealing unproven data. Dr. George F. Cahill, president of the American Diabetes Association, issued a statement regarding the theory that insulin causes blindness, mentioning that eye problems were described prior to the discovery of insulin, and that eye problems were also found in patients not on insulin. Lowenstein and Preger failed to mention that fact.

I cannot change the facts of illness, of what has happened, of what might happen.

I have chosen to deal, not with the duration of time, but the quality of the time I live in the present.

16
Regeneration

I PERFORM THE RITUAL of self-injection twice a day with a shaky faith in the power of insulin. It keeps me alive, but does not have the power to heal. Diabetes is a degenerative disease; I cannot heal my body, or the slow damage done to it. I have read that there is a high suicide rate among diabetics. I can empathize with that kind of despair, but not with that kind of action.

As I have come to an acceptance of the possibility of future incapacity, my joy in what I presently have becomes intensified. I find new value in and appreciation for life in all its wonder. What is usually taken for granted becomes magical. I would rather have ten truly productive years than fifty spent in the pursuit of petty concerns.

I wake in the morning and look out the window. In the haze, a large suspension bridge curves across the bay. I am always enchanted by the view. The simple act of seeing becomes a way of seeing.

I look at Carol, and she is more than just a woman. She is a work of art, a perfection I have been gifted to view. I realize that every day. I will never become accustomed to our marriage. I will never become bored.

I cannot imagine a day when I could lose my appreciation of the emotional and physical textures of love. I have been given that gift. Too often I forget that it is not forever, that Carol and I only have a certain amount of time, and the quality of that time is precious. Life will never become a habit because we realize the possibility of loss.

I can face the possibility of impotence because I realize I have made the most of the time I have. I have turned my pain to pleasure. That is an attitude of survival that is more valuable than any medical intervention.

If I walk in pain, I also move with the knowledge of that simple gift we too often take for granted. I live in a world of miracles most people never ponder. And because of that fact, I will never look back with regret. I no longer fear the future; I have not been punished, have not been given less. I have been blessed with acute senses. I have seen miracles.

And if I fear for my children, I am comforted by the certainty that they will know love and compassion. They will not seek physical or material comforts at the expense of humanity.

Diabetic concerns can form the basis for a valuable philosophy of living. Recognition gives way to an intensified view of living—not merely a will to survive, but the need to survive and prosper.

We have all been given gifts, but very few of us are appreciative of those gifts.

I have seen the possibility of great pain in the future. I have been given great joy in the present.

I have found myself, and I am content.